MAKE THEIR DAYS

ABOUT THE AUTHOR

Enid Portnoy, Associate Professor of Communication Studies and a Faculty Associate of the Center of Aging at West Virginia University, holds a Bachelor of Science degree in Speech communication, a Master of Arts degree in Oral Interpretation from Northwestern University, and a Doctor of Education degree in Curriculum & Instruction from West Virgina University. She is a certified AARP Reminiscence Trainer and conducts many workshops on the topic. She has taught elderhostel programs, in-service training for health providers, and special courses for lifelong learners. Her intergenerational organization, INTERGENERATE, was a recipient of a Governor's Service Award as an exemplary volunteer service organization contributing to community living in West Virginia. Dr. Portnoy's articles have appeared in both communication and aging journals. She is co-author of *Phonetically Speaking* and *Nonverbal Communication* instructional workbooks and has a chapter on "Reminiscence as Communication" in *Aging and Mental Health*, published by the Mid-America Congress on Aging. Her chapter on "The Older Woman" appears in *Cross Cultural Communication and Aging*, published by Lawrence Erlbaum Associates. She is also a member of the Eastern Communication Association and The Association for Gerontology in Higher Education.

MAKE THEIR DAYS

ACTIVITIES FOR RESIDENTS IN LONG-TERM CARE

By

ENID J. PORTNOY, ED.D.

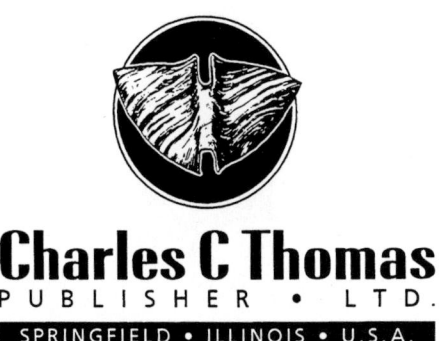

Charles C Thomas
PUBLISHER • LTD.
SPRINGFIELD • ILLINOIS • U.S.A.

Published and Distributed Throughout the World by
CHARLES C THOMAS • PUBLISHER, LTD.
2600 South First Street
Springfield, Illinois 62794-9265

This book is protected by copyright. No part of
it may be reproduced in any manner without
written permission from the publisher.

© *1999* by CHARLES C THOMAS • PUBLISHER, LTD.
ISBN 0-398-06943-3 (paper)

Library of Congress Catalog Card Number: 99-11374

With THOMAS BOOKS *careful attention is given to all details of manufacturing and design. It is the Publisher's desire to present books that are satisfactory as to their physical qualities and artistic possibilities and appropriate for their particular use.* THOMAS BOOKS *will be true to those laws of quality that assure a good name and good will.*

Printed in the United States of America
CR-R-3

Library of Congress Cataloging in Publication Data

Portnoy, Enid J.
   Make their days : activities for residents in long-term care / by Enid J. Portnoy.
     p.   cm.
   ISBN 0-398-06943-3 (paper)
   1. Long-term care facilities--Recreational activities. 2. Nursing homes--Recreational activities. 3. Aged--Recreation.
4. Recreational therapy for the aged. I. Title.
RA999.R42P67   1999
362.1'6--dc21   99-11374
                                                                                     CIP

INTRODUCTION

Communication is an activity most of us engage in every day without much conscious deliberation. It fulfills one of our most significant needs: to express ourselves in response to others. Communication is a circular process of looking, listening, interpreting and then responding. During social interactions we share both verbal and nonverbal cues.

Depending upon our personality, we may become more aware of and more comfortable with one type of communication channel (eye contact, voice sounds, facial expressiveness, etc.) over others. This, then, becomes our preferred way of creating and responding to messages. As an example, if you are more sensitive to visual stimuli, you are likely to retain "eye pictures" longer in your memory, and may find yourself repeating such things as "I see what you mean," or "I get the picture," or "Can you visualize that?" You begin to feel more satisfied if people convey messages to you using your preferred communication channel.

This book is all about communication. It provides basic insights into the various forms of the world's most common interpersonal activity, but it is much more: it also offers a wealth of specific suggestions for activities that can be used in one-on-one or group communication settings as in residential facilities for the elderly. However, activities can be adjusted for use in other settings and with other population groups. For example, intergenerational activities can be used to introduce members within a church or school or for social gatherings where people come together for effective conversations. The goal of such activities is to initiate, increase, and enhance communication and to have fun doing it!

For many tomorrows, the number of older people will be more prominent in our lives. The frail elderly will continue to move into and through our institutional care systems. They will surely make greater demands on resources, energy, and staff creativity; while their basic need for a responsive communication partner will remain strong. We would all benefit by prominently displaying on our wall this statement by Malcolm Cowley (1980) from his book, *The View From 80*:

> *To enter the country of old age is a new experience, different from what you supposed it to be. Nobody, man or woman, knows the country until he has lived in it and has taken out his citizenship papers.*

PERSONAL IDENTITY

In many long-term care facilities, there is insufficient interest to separate the personal "seed" stories that help create an older person's identity. Time, like the schoolroom's chalk, has left its mark on all of us. However, institutional living sometimes becomes a struggle for many older residents to keep their personal identity from slipping away. One way to get to know an older person is through responsive communication and recall of their past through reminiscence activity. Chapter IX provides an in-depth perspective on the very important topic of reminiscence.

Although all memories are not positive, the older person usually welcomes recall of the past. Listeners during the communication process should not prevent an exchange of negative as well as positive experiences. All are valuable in getting to know the older individual. Just as parents and teachers were early role models, later, in facilities established for the elderly, others now act as communication models and conversation partners.

Introduction

Each person's life has been compared to a daisy. What is seen outwardly (when people take the time to look) is a spoke of white petals representing the visible manifestation of the person's lifestyle and behavior. Each petal is connected to a center cluster of minute, golden seed-heads representing individual experiences. Each seed-head is distinctive, yet together represent one central image. It takes time to uncover the middle cluster, and still more time to understand how each seed-head represents an important part of the person's life experience.

The President of the Association for Gerontology in Higher Education has written, "One grows old with a history—a history of interactions across the generations . . ." (Ansello, 1991). Therefore, a videotaped record of a resident or potential resident can be encouraged. The film might include the person speaking and functioning in the home environment, and a chronological display of the past as reflected through family photographs and artifacts. Once in the long-term facility, videotape equipment could be made available to volunteers to use as a current record of the older individual and their adjustment for family members.

To assist an activity director to accomplish goals, the family, program leaders, staff and volunteers can be drawn into planning. Chapter V will explore ideas to enlarge activity support and involvement. It is said that the difference between an optimist and a pessimist is that an optimist goes to the window each morning and says, "Good Morning, God!" and the pessimist goes to the window and says, "Good God, Morning!" As people who work with the elderly, we can continue to work to find the lighter side of situations in order to brighten the lives of older people. The best way to share your activity involvement is through communication.

ACKNOWLEDGEMENTS

This book was inspired by some wonderful older people who believe in the value of communication as a creative outlet in old age. To keep them and all of us involved, I encourage you to try the activities and interaction exercises included. Involvement with others strengthens our commitment to one another at any age.

My thanks to Glenda Bixler for her assistance and encouragement.

CONTENTS

Page

Introduction   v

Chapter

1. Communicating With the Aging   3
2. Communicating a Motivational Message   11
3. Activity Starters   27
4. Family Involvement   31
5. Active Involvement   37
6. Motivating Volunteers   47
7. Nursing Home Involvement   49
8. Residents' Activity Involvement   53
9. Creative Activities Programming   57
10. Reminiscence   63
11. Intergenerational Activity   73
12. Art Activities   81
13. Drama Activities   87
14. Music Activities   95
15. Nature Stimuli Activities   97
16. After Words   99

MAKE THEIR DAYS

Chapter 1

COMMUNICATING WITH THE AGING

Age is not important unless you're a cheese.
—Helen Hayes

ADAPTATION

From the moment we are born we begin to change. Our physical self takes on a new form and in normal aging our mental capacities are waiting to be stimulated. We begin to adapt to our surroundings establishing effective behavior patterns to move us from one life stage to another. Life becomes a continual process of adaptation to change.

Confronted by a large number of diminished capacities associated with aging, many older Americans find themselves in need of extra caregiving which is most commonly handled by a female. Many women in middle or old age assume the responsibility of caring for an older relative at the same time they are pursuing a career and/or taking care of a spouse and/or their own children. It is estimated a woman will spend eighteen years of her life raising her children and almost the same length of time caregiving an older parent. This situation has led to the descriptive term, "sandwich generation." The term refers to people caught in the middle between significant others who need assistance at different stages in their lives; e.g., a female caregiver who gets squeezed between younger and older generations who need her.

When caregiving for an older person becomes excessive and is viewed as an impossible burden for any number of "good" reasons, institutional care may be considered a viable alternative. During this time feelings of guilt and obligation may accompany a reluctance to turn over the care of the person to an outside family source. Special attention must be given to ways communication can be employed to assist both the older person and others involved in the older person's care.

FIRST CONTACTS

Before the older person is placed in a new environment, he or she is often brought to the area as an aid to general orientation. Whenever the first personal interview takes place its significance cannot be overlooked. Some nonverbal researchers have suggested that the impact of an interpersonal message is communicated primarily by the nonverbal rather than the verbal cues transmitted. These cues may include the posture of a person, the type, frequency and intensity of gestures, the type and duration of eye behavior, the type of voice quality and the use of pauses displayed. In a 1955 study, Sainsbury suggested that during an interview situation, gestures of individuals increased in proportion to the level of perceived stress reactions during the communication, even though the person's body seemed to be at rest. In other interview studies when a person felt anger and depression, an increase in leg and head movements seemed to occur. These are clearly nonverbal cues that the body displays unconsciously and can reveal emotional states. Watch for such cues when an older person is being interviewed.

Facial Cues

Individuals are instructed to search for nonverbal clues in a person's face to discover their true feelings. However, nonverbal communication research also suggests that in our culture many people have learned to be facial liars. They know how to manipulate the face so that facial messages are controlled by seemingly indifferent facial expressions. Limb movements and muscular tensions in the body are often more accurate representations of a person's feelings than a face is. With older persons, poor vision may make it difficult to observe another person's face and read their emotions accurately. In addition, being placed in a wheelchair or holding on to a walker may also increase the inability to focus on a conversational partner's face.

Body Cues

The body is like a mirror. It unconsciously absorbs another person's movements and reflects our psychological responses to that person and their message. For instance, when feeling positive toward someone, we tend to incline our posture toward the person to seek more directness and a closer connection. The communication term for this is congruence or echoic posture. When we imitate another's posture, this represents a nonverbal compliment directed toward the person. In contrast, if two people's bodies have dissimilar postural displays we assume that communicators are either unresponsive to one another or sense a perceived inequality of status. Make a simple observation of two people talking together. Regard it as an opportunity to see how the posture of one person reflects a similar or dissimilar attitude toward their partner. Remember: some nonverbal cues "speak" louder than words!

The Setting

In the office setting, where communication interviews are more likely to take place, the presence of a desk often acts as a physical barrier for conversation. As an environmental object, the desk suggests the owner's power and status and therefore may intimidate the interviewee. In the presence of older persons with any appreciable sensory losses, a desk may also block their ability to understand verbal and visual feedback cues of the interviewer. The farther away the interviewer is from an older person, the harder it may be for that person to process the necessary message cues.

What is the solution? Move a chair to the side of the desk, or move completely away from the desk (a task area) into a more informal space in the office. Invite the older person to a lounge, if it is quiet, to encourage more social and informal communication. The amount of change in a person's facial and vocal expressions, the rate at which a person speaks, and the volume level of speech can measure the arousal level of an area (how stimulating the features are). Remember that each environment has the potential to stimulate a person positively or negatively.

Making people comfortable in a communication environment may also involve careful structuring of time. Part of conversation time revolves around social/polite details in order to get to know the person and his/her immediate emotional state. The remaining time is devoted to task-related information: acquiring essential information, signing papers, explaining procedures and rules, etc. Environments contribute to the ease or discomfort an older person feels when asked to participate in the conversation.

The Context

Setting the tone for any communication occurs while an initial impression is being formed. Thoughts gathered from the first person-to-person contact remain in the memory and have a significant influence on future contacts with the person. Talking simultaneously with an older person and a family member or friend makes the communication setting more complex. The direct focus of conversation needs to be balanced between parties, with more time usually given to the older person.

Occasionally we concentrate too much attention on a family member who may seem directly responsible for institutional placement and may do most of the talking. Addressing comments to that person, to the exclusion of the older person, suggests that the older person has little input into her/his own future. Unwittingly, we treat the person as a "nonperson"— an object who happens to be present at the moment. Using questions like "What does she enjoy?" or "How does he feel about socializing with others?" or "Is she able to get down to the dining room?" emphasizes the invisibility of the older person. The use of impersonal pronouns, the lack of physical directness, and attention directed toward others can produce additional stress for the elderly individual.

Time

In our eagerness to communicate with the elderly, we sometimes ask for more information at one time than they can easily process. It is easy to bombard an older person with a series of questions. ("Is it warm enough in here for you? Shall I put another blanket here? Let's see, which sweater is the one your niece brought you?") These are common examples of communication overload or projecting too much information in a short amount of time. It is far better to acknowledge the longer response time an older person needs in order for them to process information. We must take more time to structure questions and messages in such a way that the most effective response seems evident.

Bringing conversation with elderly persons to a successful close is also critical in creating positive communication experiences. Time is a precious commodity in our society. The amount of time spent in a conversation subtly suggests how much we value a communication partner. Therefore, wasting of conversational time often results in feelings of guilt and sometimes anger. Knowing the intent of every conversational exchange helps everyone use time wisely.

In order to avoid interpersonal conflicts over time management, it is usually better to inform an older person of any limits to the communication. Announce your time availability at the onset of each conversation and, if necessary, repeat your schedule again as you bring the conversation to a close.

Sharing time with someone sends a nonverbal message of caring and willingness to become involved with that person. This does not necessarily mean that you are expected to assume only one role—that of the speaker. Rather, the role of listener may be more of what the older person prefers for you. Communication is a prized activity for many older people and consists of both verbal and nonverbal messages. We can also communicate with older people by learning to share their silence.

Hearing a person speak is not necessarily engaging in open and active listening. Become aware of your own attitudes and feelings to avoid selective bias and prejudging of others. Search for cues which are not always apparent in a communication partner. When a person is engaged in active listening the focus should always be on the other person and their message, not on the response that the listener anticipates making. An effective communicator must also be an alert and responsive listener.

LAUGHTER

Laughter is a form of health improvement in conversation. Everyone can appreciate humor if a stimulus is found which tickles the funnybone. People who are humorous have a positive view of life and are individuals that people enjoy being around. When we were younger, laughter came easier and was displayed more often in an open manner. As we age, people need to be reminded to take a lighter view of their experiences.

Having a good sense of humor is positively related to mental health. It suggests a relaxed and confident person, and someone interested in capturing the attention of others. Those who use humor effectively feel good about themselves and are successful at combating the stress in their environment. Laughter helps release a person from pain by producing endorphins—the body's natural painkillers. Laughter also enhances the immune system and stimulates the circulatory system. Generally, almost every body part moves when we laugh, including the muscles of the face. The physical exercise the body receives from laughter responses provides an internal message, exercising the lungs and increasing oxygen. The comedian, Fred Allen, knew this when he said, "It is bad to suppress laughter. It goes back down and spreads to your hips." And laughter is merely one aspect of verbal communication.

In almost every setting, communication contacts occur as a result of one person deciding on a goal to accomplish by interacting with another person. Stop and consider: what type of communication contacts is commonly experienced in a social versus a health care environment? How can we make such contacts successful by knowing more about the nature of communication?

Chapter 2

COMMUNICATING A MOTIVATIONAL MESSAGE

I'm saving that rocker for the day when I feel as old as I really am.
—President Dwight D. Eisenhower

In order to get people enthused about participating in activities, communication skills of activity staff need to be effective on an ongoing basis. How we relate routinely is oftentimes more important than the skills employed to initiate activity planning. Communication that consists of both verbal and nonverbal cues is responsible for projecting a message, although nonverbal cues (tone of voice, postural changes, gestures, eye movement, etc.) appear to convey more of the meaning in a message than verbal cues do. Nonverbal cues are much more subtle and varied than verbal cues. As an example, conveying your appreciation of someone's efforts can be displayed by a smile, pat on the shoulder, walking toward the person or sitting beside them, or nodding your head—all such cues are varied nonverbal forms of the same positive message.

YOU AND YOUR VOICE

Most of us believe that *what* a person says is of greater significance than how the message is conveyed by the voice. However, the human voice has tremendous potential and complexity in communicating emotions, regulating responses from others, strengthening attitudes, emphasizing our thoughts and ideas and even presenting conflicting message cues. Becoming aware of the ways in which the voice is used can help us develop more effective communication habits. According to nonverbal research, voice cues carry significant perceptual cues to others.

Voice Qualities

A large part of one's vocal image is conveyed by a person's distinctive voice quality. Nonverbal sensitivity to such vocal color helps individuals recognize attitudes and emotions of others. Voice quality includes pitch range, tempo, volume level and changes, dialect, and articulation patterns. When listening to a person's voice, we evaluate the quality as generally pleasant or unpleasant. Then these impressions become attached to the speaker's personality.

Of all the vocal qualities that are evaluated negatively, high on the list is excessive *nasality*. Nasality in the voice produces a whining sound that becomes irritating for the listener. The general impression of a person with a nasal voice is that of a socially undesirable personality and certainly not an individual with whom you wish to converse. This quality is difficult to listen to for any length of time due to its monotonous and nonassertive associations.

The person who lets too much breath escape while speaking uses a *breathy voice quality*. It is interesting to note how gender affects impressions of a person's breathiness. A female with a breathy quality of voice is thought to be either sensual, timid or a "featherbrain." The male with the same breathy voice quality suggests an artistic or effeminate personality. For both sexes, the sound of air escaping from the voice makes the person seem weak and reluctant to take control of a situation.

Whenever tension is present in the voice the pitch usually rises. The resulting *strident quality* is negatively evaluated. A strident voice can sound authoritative for a time, but the force behind the voice and its high-pitched sound may become tiring for listeners.

A voice with an expanded carrying power is called *resonant* and has a full-bodied, amplified sound. Many older people find it difficult to sustain enough breath to produce such a vigorous tone quality. Instead, they have a *thin* voice quality which has little carrying power, and may be punctuated by short sentences and many hesitations and other nonfluencies. Our perception of a thin voice quality suggests the timid or nonassertive person, somewhat immature and emotional.

Remember that the personality perceptions a listener receives through the voice may or may not be accurate. Why, then, should we be concerned about how the voice sounds? Because other people believe these immediate perceptions, associating vocal sounds with positive or negative images about your personality.

Speaking Rate

We also have different perceptions about individuals due to their speaking rate or overall tempo. The slower a person speaks the more friendly and sociable we perceive that person to be. In contrast, a rapid speaker is thought to be cold, unfriendly, and yet, more competent than the slower speaker. Competence in a person is also viewed as a reflection of the amount of vocal variety in a voice. The more flexible the voice, the more knowledgeable the person appears to be in manipulating the vocal message. The voice quality, tempo, and variety all evoke specific impressions about an individual.

Vocal Characterizers

Vocal characterizers reflect the emotion behind words. An example of a characterizer is a bright, cheery voice that consistently lifts our spirits versus the "growler" voice which sounds dissatisfied with everything and everyone. Sighing, laughing, crying or whining as we speak are all uses of vocal characterizer emotions. As an example, sighing while speaking is considered a compliment to the listener. It is a spontaneous release of genuine emotion that suggests the speaker feels relaxed in a partner's presence. Generally vocal characterizers help the listener decide on a speaker's feelings.

Pauses

Another element that serves as a vocal message cue is the presence or absence of pauses as we speak. Most of us would prefer our speech to be continuous, with few breaks or forced hesitations of any kind to interrupt the message. When we interact with another person it makes us nervous to have to include pauses or to listen to them in excess. Research suggests that the most common use of the pause is for purposes of emphasis or reinforcement of ideas. Pauses are commonly used in conversations either before the word or idea to be emphasized, or after the idea or word is presented. Either way, the intent is to capture the listener's attention.

The most common type of pause (or nonfluency) is the repeat. It occurs when the same sound or word is used successively and not necessarily regularly. "I want to—to—tell you that—that—I—I..." If such repetitions are excessive, comprehension is difficult for the listener. When certain pauses are not filled by sounds, the result is silence. Silence often makes us feel anxious or uncomfortable. However shared silence often reinforces trust in a relationship. Older people use silence when they need more time to initiate or complete a thought. They also use the pause to gather sufficient energy to continue speaking.

Vocal Variety

In order to keep the attention of communication partners, variety must be added to the voice. Speech sounds dull and too predictable when a listener can anticipate every pitch and loudness change and every pause. A helpful pitch exercise to increase vocal variety is to hum at the lowest pitch level that feels comfortable for your voice. With the aid of a musical instrument (recorder, piano, pitch flute) move two to three steps up the musical scale from that lowest pitch, and then begin speaking or humming on that pitch. Listen to the result. Tape-record this exercise to see how natural your pitch level sounds. What you will be doing is training your ears to identify a comfortable pitch for your voice.

Next, try to exaggerate changes in pitch called inflections. Vary the pitch above and below this comfortable pitch level to add color to words and more variety to the voice. Next, listen to the overall pace or tempo of the voice as you read aloud. Try to exaggerate increases or decreases in tempo. Read some sections faster as summary statements and then slow down to describe other specific and detailed ideas.

Vocal variety encourages greater listener attention and is generally regarded enthusiastically by others. It comes as a surprise to most people to hear themselves on a recording. The sound image of your voice is seldom the same one heard on an audio recording. Therefore, it is best to wait a while before playing back the initial recording, to provide more objectivity for an evaluation. The goal of listening is to learn to recognize vocal strengths and weaknesses so communication can be improved. Senior citizens may enjoy reading aloud or reciting short passages for audio or video recording purposes so they can hear and see themselves when the tape is reviewed.

Vocal Delivery

1. Adjust your volume level for the person's comfort. Ask: "Am I speaking loudly enough?" or "Am I speaking clearly?" Rely on such feedback from listeners to adjust your volume. Do not assume all elders have a hearing problem.
2. Use a lower pitch than usual to accommodate for hearing losses in some residents. Many older persons have difficulty hearing high-pitched voices. How does your voice pitch sound? Has anyone expressed difficulty when listening to you?
3. Preview important information before sharing it. Face the person directly and suggest: "This is important for you," or "Here is the first step you will want to remember," or simply, "Please remember this!"
4. Always allow sufficient time for older persons to respond. Do not finish thoughts for them unless there is a physical or speech need that requires your assistance.
5. Never hesitate to ask for verbal feedback. Ask: "Do I make myself clear?" or "Do I sense your anger about this?" or "Shall I write this down?" By using the first person (I) when asking or replying, you invite someone to respond personally as well. Include sufficient pause time for the information to be processed.
6. Any conversational exchange can be tiring for an older person. Watch for signs of fatigue and restlessness. On the other hand, remember that older persons are usually hungry for oral communication. What they want most is to be the speaker and not a listener. Invite them to assume the speaking turn as often as possible

Voice and Personality

The voice is a personal reflection of an individual. It is important because it usually presents an accurate vocal image of a person's personality. The "ideal voice" in the United States is often described as easily understood and unobtrusive. Sufficient loudness is critical yet difficult to achieve with some older people. Whenever possible, and especially in group situations, use an amplification system for older voices. If necessary, repeat what each resident says so that others hear their message. "You are your voice" rings true only when people are sensitive to and appreciative of the richness and flexibility of this unique human instrument.

Questions Worth Considering

1. How do you think you sound to the residents under your care and to other staff?
2. How do you think vocal characteristics of certain residents influence the way others treat them?
3. Which person is apt to get the more positive response—the person with a whiny, nasal voice, or the one with a strong assertive voice? Why?
4. What kind of comments have your friends and family made about your voice?

An interesting vocal exercise can be arranged by blindfolding a person within a group and having others repeat the same message to them until the blindfolded person successfully identifies each person's voice. Variations of this kind of voice quiz are numerous. You may wish to provide a microphone for this activity.

LISTENING PRACTICE

When have you heard someone say the following: "He acts as if he were the only one talking . . ." or "She's so impatient; I know she only wants to jump in and get her two cents worth . . ." or "He's always getting ahead of me, firing questions about things that don't really matter."?

These responses are not unusual in everyday conversations. As a matter of fact, most of us think of conversation as the opportunity to speak up rather than to quiet down and listen. Many people are so busy thinking up a response to someone that they forget to be attentive. Because of this inability to sense another person's need to verbally share thoughts and feelings, individuals unwittingly seem to close off the channel for effective listen-speak-listen communication.

Some people are very anxious and this anxiety spills over into their speech habits. The amount of time they spend waiting for someone to finish speaking may be perceived as a waste of their time; therefore, they interrupt to advance the conversation. At other times the interruption may be silent rather than verbal. Their mind races ahead of the message their conversational partners are conveying. They become involved in either planning how to respond to the part of the message heard or they become easily bored waiting for the person to catch up with their thoughts. In either case, the meaning in the message is lost.

If a conversation partner responds: "Let's see, what was the last thing you said?" or "Did you mention that already?" the person may appear to be a poor listener or too easily distracted. Give the person the benefit of the doubt by reviewing what was said. If a person adds too many "ummmhmmm's," smiles too broadly, or moves limbs or posture constantly, make a mental note of the way in which the nonverbal movements influence others. Each speaker needs a responsive listener but one who seems genuinely interested and conveys that interest appropriately. Listeners should hold back their tongue and lean forward with their ears.

Silence is often the best response to an older speaker who is sharing an emotional message or seeking input on a critical decision. Many times the person just needs a sounding board. If a verbal response is requested, just restate what the person has said: "Let's go over what I think I heard you say ..." or "If I heard you correctly, you seem to feel that ..." or "What you seem to be telling me is that ..."

When a person feels tired, impatient, or bored, it is not possible to listen effectively. Listening is not easy. It takes a lot of energy and requires full concentration. If pressing demands require a shortened conversation, set a specific time when the interaction can be resumed. Then, be sure to keep that promise! Older persons look forward to participating in a communication opportunity.

NONVERBAL COMMUNICATION

The hectic pace at which we live our lives precludes our spending a great deal of time evaluating the type of impression we project to others. We also seldom evaluate why we react either favorably or unfavorably to those we meet or with whom we work. Since our culture is so verbally oriented, we need to be encouraged to pay attention to the more subtle nonverbal cues which reveal information about ourselves and our adjustment to the environment.

When we think of nonverbal communication, it is more than a consideration of other items beside the words. Nonverbal cues represent the closest expressive actions that resemble the meaning we want to project. Examples include a gesture like a clenched fist when anger is felt, or shifting postural positions when conflict begins in a situation, or raising your eyebrows when someone or something surprising appears. Several nonverbal researchers suggest that a significant portion of the meaning conveyed when communicating with others is through the use of posture, gesture, vocal tone and pausing and facial expressiveness.

Body Movements

The body represents a catalogue of moving messages. It is seldom quiet as it unconsciously mirrors attitudes we display about those around us. One of the easiest lessons learned in society is to imitate the movements of liked others. This sends a flattering message: their company is appreciated so much that we want to move like them to feel psychologically closer.

Body movements have been categorized as conveying information (informative), those performed to change other people's behavior (interactive), and those movements associated with a person's individual style communicated to someone who knows that person very well (communicative). Through posture, we reveal our feelings. When someone's company is appreciated our body imitates the other person's body position. Conversely, when feeling dislike or feeling ill at ease with a person, a listener's posture appears different from their speaking partner's. These body position changes suggest a perceived inequality in status between the individuals.

Posture is also related to spatial distancing. We draw closer to those we like and stay farther away from those we dislike. Shifting positions and increasing arm and leg gestures are other nonverbal cues that suggest tension rather than relaxation in a relationship.

Gesturing

1. Too much body movement can distract attention from a verbal message.

2. Plan to gesture toward rather than away from people. This includes them and brings them into your private space.

3. An older person's extreme lack of gestures and body movements can be a sign of depression. Watch their daily movement patterns and compare them with any drastic change in their observed nonverbal behavior.

4. Adding gestures to conversation gives older people another source from which to process the information. Gestures add clarity to a message and help to illustrate the intended meaning.

Since the body's relatively large size makes it simple to observe nonverbal actions, it is easy to neglect some of the other subtle nonverbal message cues of a smaller area—the face.

Facial Cues

The face is thought to be the richest area for the disclosure of emotional messages. After all, the face precedes us and is viewed as an easy-to-read area for revealing true feelings. Unfortunately (or fortunately), not all faces are open and truthful. There is also no one area of the face that best reveals emotions. Few people constantly disclose all their feelings. This, despite the fact that women in our society are generally regarded as more open in their facial expressiveness and men, much less so. It is society who sets down these display rules as to how visible the facial emotions of males and females are to be. Because of gender differences, sometimes it is more difficult to "read" the nonverbal message cues of men because they have learned to mask their facial displays more effectively than women do.

The over four thousand different facial expressions offer an idea as to how versatile this part of the body can be. Just as each person develops a movement style, so a person becomes identified with a characteristic facial manner of responding. When reference is made to someone as "a sad sack," we see drooping facial features and negative facial expressions as well as the heavy posture being displayed. Sadness is the emotion being projected. In another example, a so-called "glad Harry" may be due to the ever-present grin and wide-open eye expressions which suggests happiness and a light-hearted attitude.

There is a belief that the face always reflects a natural and honest feeling-state. This is not true for a variety of reasons. Many of us have been taught that to convince someone of our truthfulness, we must establish direct and lasting eye contact with him or her. Yet, facial expressions can be manipulated to suit any situation. Therefore, it is dangerous to assume that a person who looks you in the eye is always telling the truth. It may be more appropriate to observe a part of the body which people do not expect to be so closely monitored: the arms and the legs. Those areas are less subject to scrutiny and usually not guarded in the same way the face may be.

Remember: the eyes are a powerful nonverbal message channel because they signal that the person is ready for communication to begin. Dropping the eyes or deliberately avoiding looking at another person represents a reluctance to engage a person in interpersonal contact.

Expressiveness

1. Everyone enjoys seeing a pleasant-faced person. It actually makes people feel relaxed when positive emotions are projected.

2. Facial expressions add to the meaning of a message. When an older person is unable to register or change facial expressions, this may suggest a physical or mental disturbance affecting the person.

3. Women are generally more open with facial expressions than men and are thought to be easier "to read." This finding also suggests you have to work harder to observe how men versus how women feel. Avoid thinking of the passive male face as unfeeling. Our culture encourages men to *hide* their feelings while women are invited to *display* their feelings. Generally, women are also more intuitive in "reading" emotional cues of others. This is because women engage in more eye contact to evaluate others' emotions. They also use self-monitoring behaviors to compare their own and others' facial and emotional messages.

4. When verbal and nonverbal cues seem to project opposing messages, rely on the nonverbal cues. Trust non-

verbal cues more than words alone because the body's true feelings cannot be masked.

5. It is not uncommon for visual sharpness to decrease as we age. Therefore, be sure to position yourself at a comfortable distance from older persons so they can read your facial cues easily. How will you know if they can comfortably see and hear you? Ask.

6. Test yourself by posing these questions: What message have I gathered from nonverbal cues? Are forms of expressiveness (postural changes, amount and frequency of gestures, use of space) I noticed today different from those that I have noticed earlier in this resident?

Eye Contact

1. Establishing direct eye contact with someone suggests your willingness to initiate conversation. Eye contact opens up the path for beginning a social interaction.

2. Move in closer to older conversation partners and position yourself directly opposite them. It is easier for older persons to observe the exchange of nonverbal cues if they do not have to strain to see or hear others.

3. Do not talk while moving or arranging objects (fluffing pillows, opening curtains) as it could be distracting to older people.

4. First engage the other person by calling them by name. It will get and keep their attention.

BECOMING NONVERBALLY RESPONSIVE

Use nonverbal cues to show a positive interest in someone. Smiling is a welcome sign that a person is interested and responsive to another. Accompany a smile with direct eye contact and close spatial positioning. Using touch can also provoke positive responses as long as you observe the person's nonverbal response to your actions. Generally, touch makes one feel more responsive to a person and contributes to a more positive evaluation of them. With older persons observe their reactions to your touch behaviors.

For an older conversation partner, you may want to break your message into shorter sentences, pause more, and allow much more time to get their responses. Use a warm vocal tone and continually ask the person to respond to what you are saying and doing. Smiling and nodding your head in response to their speaking seems to encourage people to respond more expansively.

The more you begin to monitor your own nonverbal communication, the easier it will be to become aware of the cues of others. Women are thought to be more accurate nonverbal judges of others' emotions and more nonverbally sensitive. This is probably because women engage in a great deal of eye contact and pick up more nonverbal details than men customarily do.

In everyday conversations so many cues are being displayed in speaking and listening roles, it is no wonder we are seldom aware of their impact. Once you find yourself evaluating how you feel about a person or a situation, try to think back to the collection of "minor" details that contributed to the generalized judgment. Chances are that the majority of the images represent nonverbal cues that made a strong impression.

The body does not lie; most of the time we are simply not aware of the combination of subtle nonverbal cues that occur during communication. By observing nonverbal cues you and others display in conversation, you will notice that older people are generally more sensitive to nonverbal behaviors than most young people.

The older person's behavior is often the result of behavior displayed toward them. What is not said but nonverbally displayed appears more revealing than the words in the message itself. For instance, if directions are given with a commanding tone and relatively quickly, an older person may feel rushed and anxious to comply rapidly. To add time demands to the message creates a great deal of unnecessary stress. In order to stimulate activity involvement, notice the influence of nonverbal cues. Become a close observer of your own nonverbal behavior as well as the nonverbal responses called up from others.

Positive Nonverbal Cues to Adopt

In order to relax older residents and suggest a willingness to approach them psychologically as well as physically, consider emphasizing the following communication behaviors. While listening: lean forward toward the person, establish direct eye contact, smile, and use head nods to show your involvement in the content of their message. Such nonverbal cues suggest a direct responsiveness and the desire to share the message.

Chapter 3

ACTIVITY STARTERS

Better to remain silent and be thought a fool than to speak out and remove all doubt.
—Abraham Lincoln

Now is an ideal time to whet the appetite of your older people about programs you have planned. Communicate your enthusiasm about forthcoming activities. By selecting activities that highlight daily routines of older people, you can offer excellent choices to increase activity interest and participation. Many of the following can be accomplished without individuals even realizing that an activity has been formally planned:

Television—Join the residents in viewing a television show and then conduct a discussion or evaluation of what was observed. This can be an ongoing activity each week, working to increase participation in each session.

Tea Sampler—With a wide collection of teas, invite residents to a tea tasting. Using small cups, have them sample many different kinds to find their favorite. Ask what the flavor reminds them of. You can also bring in varied teacups and discuss the history of china and table settings, or vote to see which is the preferred design.

Costume Staff Day—Select a particular time period or style (i.e., Colonial Days, Wild West, Victorian Period, etc.) and have staff dress in that manner for the day.

Encourage staff to initiate discussion or enthusiastically respond to questions regarding the period or style of the day.

Newspaper—Join the residents in a lounge or social room and read aloud a human-interest story to them.

Conduct discussions about the people's feelings and behavior in the news. Discuss why some people respond as they do. "Create" news stories from actual events and behavior in your group or facility. This activity can begin with someone writing a short article and develop into a program for sharing news stories. It might lead to creating a resident newsletter.

"Rights" Game—Create a residents' "Rights" Bingo-type game. This is a fun way to ensure information about basic rights of residents is discussed and understood.

Bank Day—Make paper and cardboard money with large value amounts and lettering appropriate for your facility (e.g., Happy Hills $10). This money is used on the day called "Banking Day." All services and meals become *paying* events for which residents must use paper monies as tips and fees. Staff members can serve as money collectors and cashiers. Dining rooms can offer special beverages and desserts for menu fixed "play-money" prices. Special activities may include a "pay-as-you-view" videotape or movie showing, or other entertainment. If desired, choose an historical period (1900s) or a specific place (the Wild West) to create a specific time and money source for the day.

Environment Change—Rearrange one or more of your facility's public spaces—lobby, dining, or activity areas. Follow the decision made jointly at a residents and staff meeting. Redecorate these spaces for a few days through the efforts of the committee and other residents. Example: for Valentine's Day, cut out large hearts and doilies in different shapes to temporarily attach to seating areas, walls, and windows. Resident pictures may also be moved into different areas. Encourage residents to look for such changes and express opinions as to whether the change is appreciated.

Topsy-Turvy—A fun alternative to this activity is topsy-turvy day. Convert one area to look the opposite of how it usually does. Residents could be encouraged to guess how many things in the area have been rearranged. Whenever possible, encourage residents to give opinions about the changes.

Friendship Program—Discuss how friendship changes throughout life. Ask residents to create a list of three things desired in a friend:

A. Write the ideas on a piece of paper

B. Safety pin it to clothing (shirt/blouse)

C. Find another person who has one or more of the same ideas on their shirt. Ask residents to sit beside and discuss these things.

D. Each resident describes to a partner his/her best friend while they were growing up.

Smile Day—In order to encourage a positive feeling, smile day could be designated once a month. Residents and staff would be asked to use as many smiles as possible throughout the day in interactions with others. Smile stickers could be purchased to give to everyone or presented to people at designated times of the day if they admit to having smiled. This could be associated with share-a-joke or riddle programs. A smile, like good humor, is contagious. Everyone usually enjoys sharing a positive feeling so invite residents to help distribute them.

Chapter 4

FAMILY INVOLVEMENT

Happiness is having a large, loving, caring and close-knit family—in another city.
—*George Burns*

Most families of older residents would like to feel that they could still contribute to a satisfactory quality of life for their loved one, even though living apart from them now. Unfortunately, some family members may not appear as often as desired. The reason given is that they feel they have little to add to the institutional environment. If a special effort is made to involve them in specific ways, it may be possible to reinforce their self-confidence and, at the same time, demonstrate their importance in the facility's social community. Once formal activities have been introduced, routinely include family members as participants in these new events.

The formation of a Family Council consisting of as few as 5 or 6 families, or as many as 10-12 representatives might encourage more interpersonal involvement between family and residents. Generally, due to active schedules, it is more practical to have more rather than fewer council members. A set meeting once a month could be used for the purpose of disseminating information and planning special events. Someone with computer access can create an address list and a brief newsletter mailed to all the family members of residents. Programs described here can be used to encourage council members to take a more active role in activity development and implementation.

Family Image Contest—Send invitations to the family to participate in a short dessert program which emphasizes family bonding. Each resident is encouraged to have at least one family member present who supposedly bears some physical resemblance to the resident. Photographs, which suggest physical similarities of those unable to be present, are also acceptable. A panel of judges to choose the best "look-alikes" could be selected from those residents who expect no family members to be in attendance. If available, someone with a camera could capture the "winning" family and place a copy of the photograph on display. It is also possible to select several winners.

Staff Appreciation Day—This occasion offers an opportunity to express appreciation for caregivers in the facility. Residents could be involved making decorative labels or pins which staff members would wear as official hosts/hostesses. Appreciation or thank-you posters could be created for each floor which residents could sign and decorate for the floor staff. Individual cards for family caregivers could also be made. If the facility has a public address system, council members or several people from each floor could offer a brief greeting to those in attendance. Several aspects of this activity help to create close-knit teams working together. This is also an excellent time to encourage the younger members of families to assist residents in preparing the posters or thank-you cards.

Family Talent Activity—Older residents are usually delighted to point out the special talents and attributes of a family member to their aging cohorts. It is gratifying for older people to be able to share pride in their relatives. A family talent program can involve any-age relatives of residents. The entertainment might be sharing a joke or anecdote, demonstrating a recipe with pass-along samples, a display of talent, an explanation of how to create something, showing slides or movies, etc. Have residents introduce family offerings. Someone who does not have a family member present might act as the general narrator to welcome the audience and later, to thank them for coming.

Ask family members to play the piano as background music or to participate in a sing-along with the group. If unavailable at the facility, records or tapes from the local library can be used. Although the program may be brief, the major purpose of socialization between families and residents can easily be accomplished.

Eating 'Round the World—The residents' council or the dining hall staff could select a new and little-known country once a month that would become the central focus for either a day or a week's program. A nice change is provided if live or recorded music from the culture is played both at meal times and at selected times during the day. Programs could be structured around the cultural theme with travelogues and informative discussions.

A language teacher might be persuaded to offer mini-lessons in the language common to the culture. Residents could also be made aware of the specific country's map and geographic position. Ask a local travel agent to supply a few posters from the selected country to use as visual displays. Residents can mount a display of interesting items about the country, to be placed in a public area for everyone's enjoyment.

Family Travel—Plan a group travelogue by asking family members to share slides from trips. If several speakers are willing to participate, limit the number of slides for each and include 2-3 presentations at one program, and encourage the audience to ask questions.

Cultural Awareness—Since television has brought the world into our residences, there is renewed interest in other cultures. The international food theme might connect directly to countries with the ethnic background of the residents, making those persons and their families "celebrities of the month." Programs can center on remembrances of a specific cultural heritage assisted by travel posters, travel books, music, and other audio-visual aids. Local dance groups or ethnic organizations can provide folk dance demonstrations and music. Family talent may be available for a special treat.

Art Stimulation—For increased participation, attach a large section of brown wrapping paper to a wall with masking tape. This will become a mural with drawing input from anyone who chooses to use the coloring instruments placed beside it. In addition, residents can be asked to sign their artistic contributions. It may be necessary to coordinate with one or two residents to start, remembering that participation rather than talent is the most important issue. The paper can be extended or folded to accommodate numerous entries and can easily be removed when no longer needed. Projects of this kind represent a tangible symbol of involvement and achievement for both the residents and families.

Auction—Since most residents find it difficult to leave a facility as often as they might like, families or staff could be asked to find items (less than $1 in value), to be placed on an auction table for open or silent bidding. The auctioneer can be a resident, or several residents can share the task. Bids can be taken with colored paper, chips, etc. The goal of the auction could be to ensure that each resident gets at least one item. The staff can collect extra items so a sufficient number are available. After each person receives an item, the auctioneer can invite participants to comment on their items, if desired.

House Auction—Bring craft items, solicited business gifts and resident, staff, or family white elephants to auction off to the highest bidder. On that day, picnic-type box lunches could be provided in the dining hall. Residents can also be encouraged to decorate the picnic boxes a few days before to add color and interest to the activity. Family members can be invited as guests.

Chinese Auction—A different alternative to increase activity participation is the Chinese Auction. The same items (less than $1 in value) can be purchased, with a few funny or bizarre items to make it more fun. Wrapping and unwrapping adds suspense to the event. The auctioneer should allow numbers to be pulled out of a bag by participants before the auction begins. The auctioneer begins by calling for the individual who has #1. That individual may then choose any item available. The auctioneer then allows the resident with #2 to choose an item. That individual has a choice to either keep what was chosen or trade items with #1. This trading continues until the resident who had #1 chooses from any item in the room. Of course, the fun is expanded when the "unusual" items are constantly exchanged for a better item. Note: The staff may want to "claim" a funny item if it is noticed that a resident is not happy with the exchange.

Chapter 5

ACTIVE INVOLVEMENT

I do not know what your destiny will be, but this I know: The only ones among you who will be truly happy are those who have sought and found how to serve.
—Albert Schweitzer

In a long-term care facility, all staff, family, and volunteers are important. Look upon them as extra resources for ideas and energy. The attention and recognition given to each person will help to create a more personal relationship and group feeling. Sometimes, they will bring important issues to your attention because they are more directly involved with specific tasks and residents.

RECRUITING VOLUNTEERS

Volunteers are the backbone of your facility. They contribute added luster to your professional staff and bring new ideas and faces into your site. They also can make the workload easier and lend diversity to planning with a team approach to involvement. Everyone yearns for more volunteers and more effective ways to involve them. Here are some suggestions you might try.

1. Plan a community Volunteer Recruitment Day in conjunction with other service agencies and organizations. Everyone's community is different so spend some time brainstorming with long-time community residents about the partnership your facility can develop with the community. You may also wish to secure advice and information from family members of your residents.

2. Set up more than one group meeting to gather ideas about how to interest and recruit volunteers. Begin by mailing a written invitation to people selected as idea-generators. The letter of invitation should include no more than half-a-dozen questions for people to consider and discuss. Receiving an invitation to participate makes people feel their ideas are valued. If you have time, follow up the letter with a personal call to confirm attendance.

3. For the initial idea meeting, someone might volunteer a home setting that may entice more community people to attend. During the brainstorming meeting, discuss the need for everyone to share thoughts without anyone else offering an initial objection. Once people listen to others their own involvement may be increased. During the meeting, compile a list of additional names as potential recruits. You may wish to form a phone tree so those already informed about volunteering can contact new people. If possible, create a permanent committee or a titled steering board to organize an official orientation day along with a training schedule. The orientation day's events should allow time for short breaks and serving of a snack or meal to those attending. The best location for training meetings is your own facility so that people can see where they will be working.

4. The major objectives of the orientation steering committee are to establish specific goals and duties which new volunteers will be expected to learn. Select either a chair or co-chairs to be responsible for coordinating the training program. During the volunteers' training use both staff and outside speakers to provide more program variety.

5. Once volunteers are recruited, be sure to provide ample opportunities for them to report their reactions to their new duties. A steering committee member as a liaison between volunteers and the administrative staff might moderate informal group meetings convened solely for the purpose of airing feelings. If a more formal feedback is desir-

able, have a suggestion box located in a public space or seek additional written feedback via an evaluation form. Developing such a form might be another responsibility given to members of your steering committee.

Volunteer Recognition

Recognition of volunteers is an important factor in involvement. Whether you simply announce names over a public address system, put names on a bulletin board, include them in a newsletter article, or talk about their contribution in a community newspaper, explore ways to publicly commend those who service your facility. One nursing home has a competition by which residents and staff recognize outstanding volunteers. A monthly volunteer luncheon is then held, to include special entertainment. Another option is to feature end-of-year volunteer recognition picnics or parties, perhaps even "crowning" outstanding volunteers. Whatever forms of recognition you choose, publicize it well so that volunteers can work toward a heightened sense of involvement and reward.

When volunteers are clearly outstanding, extend an invitation to them to lead an activity or create a special activity that utilizes their interests. Have them enlist other volunteers to encourage a "volunteer spread" to take place. With all the responsibilities present in your facility, it is sometimes easy to overlook the role of the volunteer. Remember to always seek input from other staff and residents as to how they are responding to volunteer assistance.

Teenage Volunteers

Due to today's high unemployment conditions, many teenagers are finding it difficult to secure employment. Although health care is often listed as one of the careers to consider for the future, little specific information may be available to help young people decide whether this is an interest they might like to pursue. By contacting public and private schools and trade schools or posting public notices on community bulletin boards in malls and recreation centers, you can extend an invitation to area teenagers to serve as volunteer interns or apprentices at your facility. The term "interns" is used because many educational institutions have begun to offer academic credit for work opportunities or internships, whether paid or unpaid. Many young people prefer an internship assignment so that they can list it on their resumés.

In order to offer a broad-based experience to a young volunteer, create a partnership with an experienced volunteer who can help explain the facility and programs. Encourage them to interact with residents, perhaps selecting two or three individuals to communicate with in a more personal manner. This may make it easier for young volunteers to get to know directly some of the personalities and needs of your residents.

PLANNING YOUR MESSAGES

Volunteers must be persuaded that there are advantages to their service. The way we motivate volunteers to become involved is often dependent upon how we communicate our message. Encourage volunteers and other staff to evaluate their own communication habits. How much enthusiasm are they able to generate? Energy is contagious. People get excited when they hear and see verbal and nonverbal cues suggesting positive involvement from others.

Allow some thinking time to plan how you are going to address volunteers and others with whom you work. All communication has the potential to create a positive response in others, particularly when we consider the "audience." Plan your communication as carefully as a

Active Involvement

politician does when interacting with constituents. Most of the time the goal is the same: to convince the audience that there are advantages to be gained from believing in the program.

With volunteers ask yourself: what is it about their age and previous background experience that can help to draw them into a circle of involvement? In biblical terms, involvement suggests a way to encircle others by bringing them into the fold of our attention. How can you plan to do this? Often the difference between what we think motivates others and what they believe to be their needs and interests separates rather than involves us.

The benefits of involvement should be constantly emphasized. Be flexible about additional benefits that can be adapted to your facility. From the verbal responses of your volunteers, past and present, compile a small pamphlet or one-page flyer directed at volunteers, which describes the benefits from participating. Examples of benefits could include:

1. An opportunity to contribute to the lives of others
2. Practical application of people's skills and talents to assist others
3. Exposure to an age group which, with a little luck, we will join one day
4. Increased cooperation and teamwork
5. Development of new relationships and interaction skills
6. Testing of one's flexibility and adaptation to new situations and personalities
7. Reflection or projected image of one's association with aging

Involvement at any age encompasses all these ideas and offers many lasting rewards. Volunteers who have successful adaptations to aging are those who have varied interests, are people-oriented, and are willing to adjust to different situations, including volunteerism.

THE KEY

While each group of activities can be adapted to suit the different needs of residents and residential facilities, the key to creative programming often lies with a well-trained and imaginative program director. If your facility does not have access to a permanent individual with program responsibilities, it may still be possible to work with volunteer help. An educational institution or social service agency may be looking for placement situations for students and interns, so people can associate their theoretical knowledge with direct practical experiences.

Consider applying for a mini-grant to help you secure training funds for people who would like to volunteer but need financial support for on-the-job training. Regional and national aging organizations often conduct workshops, short courses, and seminars in the area of programming. Contact them or use library resources to become aware of additional educational opportunities of this nature. By combining forces with other types of elder organizations and residential settings in your area, several facilities can have rotating programs for everyone's benefit.

Staff Involvement

The following ideas can generate discussion or stimulate staff involvement:

1. Encourage staff to cut out calendar activities that can be placed on the "plan of care." Aides cannot be expected to look at the larger calendar of activities, but they can be encouraged to remember items in individual care plans.

2. Emphasize how important aides and volunteers are in your facility and find ways to compliment them, especially in the company of residents.

3. Plan activities linking nurses and aides together in activity work and in social events in your facility.

Active Involvement

4. Remind staff that when aides are involved in activities, others can relax and not be solely responsible for activities or residents.

5. When dealing with disturbed patients or Alzheimer's patients, one-to-one activities often work best. Be aware of rapid shifts in attention span and plan short activities or ones that will not be destroyed by patients wandering in and out.

6. Whenever possible offer choices of activities. Be flexible enough to drop one activity to pursue another more appropriate one for what may be going on.

7. Remember: some participation in comparison to none at all is better in terms of residents. Do not be discouraged if some residents seem more reluctant to participate. Encourage their attendance even if they choose to be silent observers.

8. With confused patients, it is not possible to recognize how little or how much input the person is receiving from an activity. Their presence at an activity, although passive, may still prove meaningful for their stimulation.

9. The more familiar something is the more it will appeal to everyone in some way. Example—If you work with old hymns that people have heard for a number of years, they are more likely to react positively to the activity associated with it. Pair the familiar with your new activities.

10. Patients with disabilities may require more detailed planning on your part, but stimulation and participation may make a critical difference for their emotional and physical well being.

11. An activity leader and volunteers must appear energetic and positively involved in every activity. You are the role model. What you do and how you do it significantly affects the enthusiasm transmitted to residents.

12. Choose different resident leaders or staff volunteers for activities. This strategy can add sufficient variety to make an activity seem new. Encourage staff to comment on residents' participation.

13. Remember to ask staff members for activity ideas. The more ideas received, the more choices there are to select. The staff members with "winning" ideas can be given a reward (free lunch, certificate, prize ribbon, etc.).

14. Invite staff to come up with talent show entertainment. If successful, this could be an ongoing program.

15. Challenge staff of nearby facilities to participate in team sports, or exchange talent programs, or plan contests for the most creative activity programs.

16. Have staff be responsible for a "Dessert Surprise." Staff must cook or bring in desserts to share with residents, along with a panel of resident judges to evaluate them.

17. Encourage staff to write biographical entries on individual patients and staff experiences. These can be character sketches, or topics like "The funniest situation here," or "The most inspiring situation," and "Something I will never forget here." These can also be printed, put on a bulletin board or newsletter or the best ones read aloud.

18. Have joint staff-resident activity programs like bowling, aerobic-type exercising, etc.

19. Joke of the week contest. Staff can write up a joke and then tell it over the P.A. system or in the dining room as part of a program. According to residents' laughter or applause, a winner (or winners) is selected.

20. Take time to uncover talents and hidden skills of staff. Rewarding their talent can create much good will.

21. When special awards are to be presented to staff, invite their families to the program. Selected residents can act as hosts/hostesses for guests. Community officials can also be invited to attend "recognition days" to reinforce public appreciation for effective workers and their contributions.

22. Use a facility newsletter or bulletin board to print short biographical sketches of staff and volunteers. A resident who likes to socialize or enjoys writing can be asked to interview different individuals.

23. Although it may not seem original, place a suggestion box in a public space where staff and volunteers are invited to write any comments and improvement suggestions. Usually this is done anonymously. Later on, use the idea as discussion starters at staff meetings, print or post them, or ask for others to comment further. This strategy provides an open communication channel in your facility.

24. An after-hours social for all staff is another idea worth considering. Keep a part of the program a surprise and plan some type of appreciative recognition for them.

25. A "secret pal" partnership between staff and residents can be encouraged with the recognition announced on a specific day.

Videotaping

The video camera has become a common household item. Any activities in your location can be videotaped for future viewing and program sharing, if you first secure written permission of the residents. A *visual* record of programs, as on videotape, is an effective orientation tool for outside individuals considering your facility as a potential resident or volunteer and who wants to evaluate its activities. Videotaping can also be used by family members to prepare a personal documentary of present residents or those individuals on the waiting list for your facility.

Share a Life

The program or residence director and the staff need to know the life history interests and experiences of residents, in order to match them with program objectives. The more knowledge the staff has about the residents the easier it is to approach them in an individualistic and humanistic manner. Communication skill development should be routinely addressed to ensure effective participation by staff. Providing an overview of communication will emphasize, as well as enhance, the skills necessary for ongoing interaction.

Elders with special needs can benefit from creative programming. Mentally retarded individuals have increased their communication opportunities and enhanced their self-image, as a result of interactive programming. Residential care creative programs can provide an outlet to integrate this special population into activities designed to develop the expressive potential of all elderly residents.

Chapter 6

MOTIVATING VOLUNTEERS

If a person is called to be a streetsweeper, he should sweep streets even as Michelangelo painted, or Beethoven composed music or Shakespeare wrote poetry. The person should sweep streets so well that all the hosts of heaven and earth will pause to say, here lived a great streetsweeper who did his job well.
—Martin Luther King, Jr.

One of the best ways to gain volunteer help is by sending representatives of your facility to speak before community and church groups. If there is a volunteer section in your local paper, advertise an open house or informational meeting. Contact a college social work or gerontology department to ask for help in recruiting volunteers. Posters downtown and in malls can also be excellent publicity calls for volunteers. In addition, an active resident family council can help to write or telephone officers of area clubs and organizations, asking them to announce a volunteer call at their next meeting. The organization list can be secured from the Chamber of Commerce.

In groups (staff, families, residents, etc.), discuss the importance of motivation and how we get others involved in facility programs. Here are direct suggestions:

1. Ask people who volunteer to share two or three "significant accomplishments" made during the previous or current week in your facility.

2. Put these accomplishments on a flip chart, board or poster for public display.

3. Decide on a tangible reward of some kind (certificate, free lunch, etc.) for the most effective volunteer activity suggestions, or the most effective volunteer(s).

4. Announce volunteers of the day, week or month over a P.A. system.

5. Announce a volunteer motivational goal for a specific time period on the P.A. system or a bulletin board so that everyone strives toward a specific goal.

6. Use agreed-upon motivational goals to establish group discussions for meetings and evaluation sessions. Program and volunteer evaluations can be both informally or formally conducted. Be sure you include some kind of evaluation for each volunteer activity.

7. Always thank your volunteers for any degree of participation. Address people by name. If you cannot recall names, create volunteer badges that are a form of identification and recognition.

8. Present special awards or certificates for the "Best Motivational Ideas" of the month (or time period decided upon).

Remember: Staff are always "on stage" modeling the best behaviors and motivating others by their attitudes. Delivering the "call to participate" is as important as the message itself.

Chapter 7

NURSING HOME INVOLVEMENT

Worry is like a rocking chair;
It gives you something to do but doesn't get you anywhere.
—Anonymous

Almost everything we do in the long-term care facility can be attributed to our ability to gain the support of others, in order to fulfill our roles and responsibilities toward residents. The cooperation of others is the key element in determining how effective programs and relationships with others can become. Involvement is a given; however, having the staff, sufficient volunteers, and family involvement does not automatically predict resident involvement. Emphasis on communication concerns from the time of the first interview continues through get-together activity starters with families, staff, and volunteers. The emphasis must be on ideas to strengthen interpersonal connections within the facility.

INVOLVING RESIDENTS

How many times have you been frustrated with the half-hearted response you receive from residents about personal or program involvement? Someone may be too tired to participate, not interested in an activity, doesn't feel up to joining in an activity, etc. Although you may take such comments as a personal affront, there are some strategies that can encourage people to come into your circle of involvement; after all, the reason for program activities is to *"Make Their Days!"*

Select certain residents to be "gatekeepers"—individuals who have more perceived status with others and can serve as a role model to interest others and affect their behavior. By spending a little extra time interacting with and training these key people you can reinforce their competence. This is also a good way to get them to develop a greater sense of responsibility toward a volunteer project or planned activity.

Referent Power

Communication research suggests that in order to persuade someone, referent power is important. The term suggests using a person who is respected as a motivating force and whose reactions and evaluation of behavior is personally meaningful. The person's perceived attitude makes individuals want to please them and do their best.

To apply that to the role of staff or volunteers, when a warm relationship with residents is developed, they are more likely to want to please and therefore comply with requests to participate. "I like you and therefore, I want to do what you ask of me." A team approach to get others involved is a must; seeing the interest exhibited by both staff and volunteers represents a stronger appeal for residents. Even though it takes extra time to inform others of motivations and ideas for activities and socialization, the minutes spent will reap long-term results.

Involving Others

Assigning important duties to selected residents can also involve others. If the task one person has will significantly affect the success of an activity (and you emphasize this) most people will take pride in contributing their expertise. "Betty will pass out the cards tonight, and John, can you be responsible for arranging the piano bench and light for our guest? I have asked Margaret to select the first song we will sing." Recognizing people publicly is another way to display your appreciation for their involvement.

Recognition and Reward

Every kind of resident involvement can be acknowledged in some way. If outside guests are visiting your facility, assign certain residents the roles of host-hostess and present them with a special badge or identification ribbon to wear for the day. When an activity begins, remember to acknowledge by name those residents that are involved in both the planning and implementation of it. For any residents who attend the most activities within a prescribed time (i.e., a month or three months) a special certificate can be presented. Recognition can also be given to those who attend and act as helpers with other residents who may not be as physically or mentally able as others.

In this age of word processors, it takes a short amount of time to create your own certificate, print it and make multiple copies for use on different occasions. You can even use certificates as an art activity. Encourage residents to decorate the certificates in different ways for specific occasions.

Different types of rewards for residents' involvement can be created from residents' suggestions. You might have a contest for the best involvement ideas to reward residents. Decorate a suggestion box in the hall and have blank paper and an attached pencil available. See what kind of ideas residents contribute. You will have lost nothing even if the number of ideas is small. If you do adopt a resident's suggestion, the "winner" might also be rewarded. A more elaborate reward system might include the creation of a point system, which could be displayed on a bulletin board. Residents could gain points for active participation, attendance, assisting the leader or others, coming up with new ideas, etc.

Residents who appear to enjoy taking on a leadership role and those who are eager to communicate their feelings to others could be organized into a mini-speakers' bureau. Their names and preferred topics could be distributed to community sources—schools, libraries, and civic organizations—as potential program speakers or panelists. Those residents could meet periodically for discussions and listen to each other's views on such topics as successful aging, retirement and its effects, nursing home lifestyles, lessons from the past, values in long-term friendships, etc. Too often, we have an imbalance of participation in an activity involving our residents as an audience for people coming into our facility. In too many instances little effort is made to send residents outside to community groups to speak or participate in other programs.

Continually seek resident feedback, both informally (talking to individuals and small groups) and formally, (asking for written suggestions, evaluation forms). Resident council meetings are not the only source to gather suggestions for motivating others. People feel more comfortable about where they work and live if they feel they have some input and involvement as to what goes on there which affects their well-being.

Cautions

The danger in relying on our own program ideas is that they are personally biased, representing personal preferences and ideas. Some ideas may not be as suitable as we think they are for the residents. It is easy to fall into the trap of shutting out others whose input may change the things we plan. Little joy and much added stress can be added when you become "The Everything Person" in your facility. An everything person is the individual who feels responsible for 110 percent of the involvement which occurs. To paraphrase the words of Mrs. Levi in the play, *Hello Dolly*: Involvement is like manure; you have to spread it around!

Chapter 8

RESIDENTS' ACTIVITY INVOLVEMENT

It's not that I'm afraid to die; it's just that I don't want to be there when it happens
—Woody Allen

Varied and stimulating activity programs go a long way to combat the isolation and lack of interaction in nursing homes. Without sufficient opportunity for socialization, a nursing home resident can lose a primary instrument of their expressive selves. Residents use both spoken language and nonverbal behaviors to adapt to their environment and attempt to satisfy needs which may not be met.

Isolation, whether social, physical, or psychological, is debilitating for older people. It's bad for people of any age and in long-term care it hinders adjustment and decreases self-esteem and the desire for independent actions. Activities that have social interaction as their goal can encourage residents to become more involved with others. Like other forms of exercise, communication and socialization improve with practice.

DIFFERENT PERSONALITIES

Those residents who use extremes of communication (who talk too much or too little) are often ignored, or perceived as people who break traditional standards of behavior. Unfortunately shy individuals may be thrust into more of an isolated state because of their reluctance to behave as though they welcome communication from others. Sensitivity in programming can be encouraged by creating different ways to pair individuals for short activities, or by having an experienced, outgoing person assist someone less experienced or sociable. Find ways to pair a talkative person with a good listener and sometimes each person begins to slowly resemble the other. Try to increase the occasions where outside visitors come into your facility and meet your residents. Working with small groups initially to bolster their esteem and provide communication can often encourage individuals to take on more active roles.

ACTIVITY VARIETY

Contrary to some popular opinion, the tried, tired and true bingo games, lectures from outsiders, movies and simple crafts are not activities which necessarily encourage interaction between residents. Small group activities, shared leadership, performing "public" speaking, dramatizing ideas and emotions and sharing reminiscences can promote more active involvement among residents.

Examine the spatial arrangement of furniture in a facility's public spaces. Does the arrangement help or hinder socialization between individuals in the facility? Take a few minutes to actually tune in on the frequency, intensity and variety of noise present in different areas. What can be done to provide a more comfortable and calm environment? There is nothing more disturbing than to have an activity interrupted because of excess noise, physical discomforts provided by the environmental features in a room, or unnecessary barriers that could have been anticipated.

Whenever possible, introduce activities with music well suited to the mood to be created. Music consists of a pulse or beat that captures a physical sense of expression. Select the right music and residents will become motivated to participate in an activity.

Learning new things by older persons may be approached with caution for a number of reasons. First, they may be fearful that they cannot perform appropriately or correctly. They may feel there is more risk involved than that they are ready to take. The desertion of familiar activities may leave them with too strong a feeling of anxiety. For many older people what is familiar is more secure and predictable. Just as younger people have varied abilities and personalities, so, too, do the elderly. Past experiences with a particular type of activity often color their desire to participate.

MOTIVATING OTHERS

Once basic needs of safety and well being are satisfied, the desire to extend our social selves surfaces. Building self-esteem is often emphasized as an objective for many activities with older people. To provide a responsive and stimulating environment is an ongoing goal for activity programs. The more choices, the more likelihood that the older person will decide to become involved in activities.

Just as patients rely heavily on their judgments of the health professional's communication skills to encourage them, so the activity director is seen as either a competent or incompetent stimulus for personal and task motivation. When activity directors are enthusiastic, people are more likely to try to please them by imitating their attitude. Older people often desire to express their personal appreciation of the director by involving themselves in the scheduled activities.

Everyone enjoys being around someone with a positive attitude. The spillover effect is pleasurable and adds to a person's sense of acceptance and well being. Too often activities are predictable and planned along traditional themes; there are few opportunities to break out of familiar scheduling to create an innovative program. We know from research as well as anecdotal examples, that humor and laughter are both healthful and energizing. When something is fun to do, it becomes easier to believe in its benefits and convince others to get involved.

Identify resident links (people) who will assist with an activity. Develop a good relationship with aides and other staff. Encourage them to support activities and offer feedback. Recognize their contribution to serve as an additional incentive for activity involvement. Don't forget to be patient. Remember: "Grass, in time, becomes milk!" and enthusiastic and creative activity directors become outstanding role models for everyone.

Chapter 9

CREATIVE ACTIVITIES PROGRAMMING

The older we get, the better we were.
—Anonymous

Creative programming for adult residential care continues to be an important need. Although programming may vary, the basic goal should remain constant: to offer an opportunity for interaction and stimulation for all residents. Strong programming can help to promote both the mental and psychosocial health and well being for older residents. Creative program activities can also offer residents in varied contexts such as day treatment programs, board and care homes and congregate housing new perspectives and communication opportunities in order to help them express feelings which may have been muffled by the perceived impersonal nature of their setting.

Criticism has often been leveled against the lack of stimulation offered to residents within large residential-care settings. Without opportunities to exercise the mind as well as the body an older person may not adjust to the surroundings successfully. The human need to share thoughts and feelings with others does not decrease with age. On the contrary, older residents often express the desire to have additional opportunities to contribute to social interactions and to bolster their self-esteem through shared communication.

The best type of activity program is one which requires involvement (mental and/or physical) from all participants. Unfortunately, too many activities reinforce passive acceptance from residents and contribute little stimulation to the communication environment.

Activities are only limited by the imagination. And to provide assistance, the remainder of this book provides a number of activity descriptions that may be used or adapted for older people. Emphasizing a single activity or combining one or more can increase variety. Activity suggestions have been grouped by topic in the following chapters to allow easy reference. Two favorite programs—Reminiscence and Intergenerational—are described in detail and can be easily adapted and/or implemented in most facilities. Consider discussing activity ideas with a few residents to evaluate their initial reactions. By doing so, it gives you a mini-support group who can encourage others to actively participate. To explain the directions for any of these activities, proceed one step at a time. Older people are often distressed by "communication overload" (presenting too much information to them at once). It is also better to give a demonstration before launching an activity. Reassure individuals that the first run-through of an activity is for practice purposes, only. Some people who initially decline to participate may be more willing to do so once they see how simple it appears to be. Using positive verbal "strokes" to motivate all residents is another reassuring technique.

GETTING STARTED

A simple activity that stimulates the mind and requires few "extras" involves category word associations. An individual in the group is asked to choose an alphabet letter and announces it to everyone. Someone else selects one category (e.g., desserts, flowers, cars, and holidays). Then each person's task is to think of several items in the category that begin with the chosen letter. For example, "Let's see how many foods you can think of that begin with an 'L'." This exercise can be connected with movement or art by asking residents to draw some of the category objects and then demonstrate their function. Try pairing residents so that people who seem to have quicker responses may assist those who have more difficulty coming up with associated words.

Studies suggest that some older people are often unable to encode stimuli, recall names, or use verbal mediation. Yet other forms of expression (i.e., art, music, and movement) other than initial verbalization can be introduced for programming variety. Two or more nonverbal expressive forms can be combined in the following manner: a mood-appropriate classical music selection is introduced at the same time each resident is given drawing paper and the choice of a colored drawing utensil. Since many residents continually express the desire to return "home," ask them to draw any area of the identified home place they recall. It does not matter how artful the final result is; all that matters is that they concentrate and try to sketch some semblance of a physical space (i.e., a bedroom, a closet, kitchen area, the attic). Keep the music on until everyone in the group completes the drawing. At that time, invite them to share their drawings, explaining some detail of the picture and describing a specific event that took place. Then, initiate a discussion about the people associated with that space. Ask how they felt as the drawing was created, and how much they remember about their feelings at the time. This activity usually produces a wide variety of stories that can encourage others.

To add movement to the activity, ask participants to imitate the way that someone or something (e.g., animal, tree, and play item) moves. Strive to include both vigorous and gentle movements in beginning exercises. Placing emphasis on one area of the body at a time is often easier for residents' concentration and physical flexibility. Waving scarves or moving balloons encourages participants to imitate the shapes and rhythmic pattern of objects.

Movement exercises also have the potential to enhance the self-image of residents. The natural environment surrounding the residence can serve as the stimulus for calling attention to nature and changing movement patterns. Bring in natural objects, such as leaves, to demonstrate the way they are shaped and to encourage touch orientation and closer observation.

As formal programs are developed, the following overall guidelines may be useful:

• Make elder residents the hosts/hostesses for community meetings and groups in your facility. This helps to increase self-esteem and expand the role of residents.

• Residents can help plan and create an In-Service for Administrators to educate the administrators and directors about activity directors' concerns. Those who participate in activities are often the best teachers.

• Put appropriate activities for each patient on the care plan which aides and volunteers use constantly.

• Make sure the aides know that the type and quality of residents' attendance will be used for evaluation of programs and for accountability concerns in your facility.

• The Resident Council can vote on the most effective aids each month to offer them more staff participation incentives.

• Don't forget social isolates, bedridden patients and those unable to participate in group activities. The key word is *adaptation* in programming: create activities for smaller, special target individuals just as you do for larger, more mobile groups. Family members, if trained, can often help to implement activity ideas.

• Be alert to special media presentations that can be meaningful to your residents. Often, we read or observe media content but do not follow-through on any discussion or evaluation of the material. Discussion stimulates mental activity and reveals residents' reactions and their perception of information received.

- Residents' socialization and communication need practice opportunities. Are activities organized with sufficient time for residents to become "active" mentally, orally, and physically?
- Remember: you are only limited in your activity planning by a lack of imagination. Very often the best ideas come from a brainstorming session with others.
- Volunteering is the direct path that leads to involvement. The more people are involved in activity programming, the more they will feel responsible for significant contributions to the lives of your residents.
- Keep a log or idea journal and note ideas, thoughts and suggestions for activities and involvement. Date all entries and indicate resource people and places you can refer to in the future.

Chapter 10

REMINISCENCE

Life can only be understood backwards,
but it must be lived forwards.
—Anonymous

Health professionals, social service workers, writers and many others have documented the importance of engaging in reminiscence during our lives. The term reminiscence refers to the recall of memories, pleasant and unpleasant, of meaningful periods in a person's life. To be human is to have a multilayered web of stories that position us in time and space. The narratives we spin, which call forth images of ourselves, offer a view of our psychological and social identities. To share such stories with others brings listeners close to our significant experiences and thus reveals more about us. Robert Coleman (1974) differentiates three types of reminiscing: simple reminiscing (recalling the past, as in storytelling and anecdotes), informative reminiscing (calling up facts and details such as events, relationships, or background material), and life review (evaluating the past to bring a sense of holistic balance and peace to the present). Older citizens often engage in this last type, life review. Marc Kaminski, the co-director of the Myerhoff Center of New York City, has called a person's life review "the construction of a self they wish to be remembered by" (1991). Reminiscence has been divided into three major categories:

• Informative: making inquiry about the past to discover facts and information which the listener wishes to know;

• Evaluative: exploring specific memories in order to assess their contribution to the person's life;

- Obsessive-compulsive reminiscing: the constant reiteration of the same memory or memories because of something unresolved about the person's acceptance of them.

It is thought that old age gives one the license to use leisure time in self-reflective activities. Since we are all storytellers, the more we rehearse and repeat our stories, the more we come to believe them. The philosopher, Erik Erikson used the term "generativity" to describe the desire many older people have to provide guidance through storytelling for the next generation. Grandparents often report feelings of regret about the lack of opportunities to convey information to younger family members about their personal stories and extended family history.

As the older person reviews the past, they may attempt to resolve inconsistencies that arise. Whether the recall of the past is done silently in the person's mind, aloud in the form of a dialogue exchange with others, or in writing or recording past narratives, the simple recall of the past presents each person the opportunity to reconsider and in some cases recast the past.

Although we tend to recall activities and events much more readily than people, it is often the people (associated with those activities) and our relationships with them that usher a host of emotions into the present. As May Sarton has written, "People we love are built into us" (1977; 135). Barbara Myerhoff has elaborated on this idea, speaking of remembering as "calling attention to . . .one's own prior selves, as well as the significant others who are part of the story" (Myerhoff, 1982; 111).

Recalling our behaviors offers us the opportunity to justify them. Time is the great leveler, giving us ample reflective moments for evaluating the past. The richness of the mind's inner pictures can also entertain the reminiscer, as well as work to maintain self-esteem, fill time, resolve pain and grief, help with adjustment to losses, connect past accomplishments to a sense of personal worth, and provide companionship and opportunities for increased communication.

Such memories of the past can be aroused spontaneously or invoked intentionally, with the help of planned stimuli. These stimuli may take the form of visits to former familiar areas, old photographs or correspondence, well-remembered pieces of music, familiar scents, etc. In social work with older adults who have mental problems, memories are sometimes invoked for their therapeutic benefits.

PROGRAMS FOR OLDER ADULTS

In my own work, I design, conduct, and study activity programs for older adults at nursing homes. These programs use reminiscence techniques for both therapeutic and recreational aims, and often yield positive results. In one program, two high school students were paired with one senior citizen to tape record reminiscences of the senior citizen's teenage years. From the extended interviews, one narrative was chosen to be published in a book of selected senior citizen memories, recast by the students as a creative writing exercise. The book was then used as the trigger for further intergenerational reminiscence discussions among the seniors.

In another project, a costumed narrator introduced the history of the seventeenth century to residents of four different nursing homes. As she described daily life during that time period, she passed out reproduction museum artifacts she had brought along, including clothing, candles, tools, and familiar household items which residents were encouraged to handle. A lively discussion developed as individuals recollected experiences with similar objects in their past. Childhood was a common focus of the stories, and certain individuals who were usually withdrawn, talked with animation during these programs.

Another activity mentioned earlier is especially appropriate to initiate reminiscence. Groups have been led through a guided imagery exercise in which participants recall memories of "the home place." Each person is told to visualize the one particular area where she or he was most comfortable, and then, narrated by the leader, each reflects silently on the visual and sensory details of that place.

Senior citizens may be asked to recite from memory poetry they learned as children, in order to discuss early school days and to reenact events and activities from early life through role-playing. One group developed an outline for a play on one-room school houses and presented it for several outside groups. Because the players generally improvised the script, new stories were continually added that reflected shared history of both players and audiences. Such experiences bolster self-esteem and feelings of accomplishment for many of the participating seniors.

Our Personal History-Making

Why do we all engage in looking backward and reminiscing throughout our lives? Why are programs that stimulate memories so effective and enjoyable? At least part of the reason is our desire for self-control. Sometimes it seems that in times past we have been more able to exert independence, to actively manipulate events and relationships than we are able to do in the present. One's personal history making, a highly creative process affords the chance once again for such control. Through reminiscing, we can review what has happened in the past, evaluate what changes we might make, and present ourselves to ourselves as well as to others. Given their importance, perhaps we should spend more time examining the personal history stories that make up our lives.

Sharing Memories As Therapy

During the aging process, we may look around us and agree with Wordsworth that "The world is too much with us . . ." For some older persons there is a tendency to want to psychologically escape from present problems by finding comfort in contemplation of the past. Reflection on earlier times when we were able to cope better seems to create a sense of well being.

Research suggests that, for the elderly, long-term memories are more easily called to mind than short-term memories. Reevaluating details from the past is an easier task than recalling events from recent moments. It is possible that too much reliance on the past may even encourage a lack of awareness about present-day attitudes and situations.

As pointed out in the book, *Helping Relationships: Basic Concepts for the Helping Professions*, by A. Combs, *et al.* (1972), "When a person looks back at some event in the past, what he remembers is not what really happened but that event colored by the meaning it had for him then and has now. He remembers what seemed to him at the time was happening, or even more inaccurately, what it now seems to him must have happened. The memory of an event is thus a belief about it, not an accurate record of it."

This subjective coloring can provide communication clues as to the person's value system. Many older persons are regarded as traditionalists in their thinking and behavior: they rely on the past as the sole source of authority and wisdom. "I was smarter in those days." "My father would have known how to talk to a man like that." "We knew how to control people in that situation." The process of recounting the past becomes a significant part of oral sharing for older individuals.

By communicating meaningful past experiences, a social connection is formed between parties. As Martin Buber tells us in "The Word That is Spoken" from the book *The*

Knowledge of Man (1965), "The importance of the spoken word is grounded in the fact that it does not want to remain with the speaker. It reaches out toward a hearer, it lays hold of him, it even makes the hearer into a speaker, if perhaps only a soundless one."

Recounting the past may bring about more of an objective perspective to an individual's needs and thoughts. Each person becomes a partner to help another construct her/his own reality. Often that responsibility is invoked simply by being present as a sympathetic listener. In every stage of the life span, humans experience a social need to communicate. Unfortunately, as we get older, many of those with whom we prefer to interact are no longer available to us. Physical separation and death take our most valued partners from us. The social circle of the older person narrows and unless we make a conscious effort to expand it, communication opportunities decrease.

Sharing memories with others is a way to share a part of us. When we communicate with an older person, we engage in a valued activity that is also viewed as a positive message of interest in the individual. Open and responsive reactions during the interaction help to reinforce the message that the older person is a significant "other." Information that is shared about the past becomes a comforting foundation for the development of a mutually satisfying communication relationship between the narrator and the listener.

Smell and Memory

Of all the senses, smell is one of the most direct communication channels linked to memory. The section of the brain that identifies odors lies very close to the area that controls emotive memory. When we are aware of a smell message it is often accompanied by a specific emotional memory. In his work at the Monell Chemical Senses Center in Philadelphia, Dr. Barry Lyman has discovered that odors attached to individual people, settings, and time are more likely to stimulate specific memories. The link between memory and smell is forged because we subconsciously process our orientation to a place and a person with those scents that permeate the environment at that moment.

Researchers at the Monell Chemical Senses Center suggest that pleasant odors appear to elicit happy memories while unpleasant odors invite unhappy ones. At Yale University, researchers found that apple-spice and lavender scents create positive responses: apple-spice can reduce blood pressure if people are stressed and also seems to avert panic attacks, while lavender makes subjects more alert (Yale Researchers, 1987).

When talking with residents, specific smell memories can be used for sensory recall activities. Residents can be involved in making smell sachets using scented cotton balls or small bags filled with different smell stimuli. In order to stimulate olfactory memories, heavily scented objects should be used with older persons as they may have a smell deficit or some form of cognitive impairment due to the aging process which requires sharper sensory input. Scented items can also be placed in small boxes or individual plastic bags for distribution. Each box or bag should have a small, identifiable sniff hole through which the odor can be detected.

Questions Worth Thinking About

The program area of Reminiscence is viewed as holding great promise. Reminiscence has been used as a form of therapy, as well as a communication tool. There is a natural tendency for elders to look back to their past as a time more control and self-satisfaction was exercised than in their present situation. Consider:

- What opportunities do your residents have to reminisce? Is there a program offered which encourages reminiscing?
- What opportunities do the mentally impaired have to reminisce in your facility?
- Do you spend more time communicating with the mentally intact than you do with the mentally impaired?
- What experiences do you share with your residents? Do you share these equally with those who are mentally impaired?

Research suggests that people who have had a rich imagination throughout their lives will be predisposed to continue such introspection as they get older. Remembering events from one's past in order to integrate and resolve conflicts can result in higher degrees of life satisfaction and a more positive self-concept. Individuals who spend time trying to evaluate their past often seem to have a healthier outlook on how to adjust to stressors in the present.

The act of reminiscing often functions as a time filler for older people. Moments spent recalling the past help individuals to fill the "empty moments" of the present. However, if the experience is intrapersonal (i.e., the person engages in solitary reflection), there is a danger that unpleasant situations and unresolved conflicts may take on even larger proportions in the person's mind. It seems more beneficial to share reminiscence with one responsive listener or with an audience of interested persons. When a listener displays an accepting and open attitude, the message sent is that the speaker's feelings have value. Even people suffering from depression may be helped by an involvement in reminiscence as well as with validation techniques.

Program leaders in either a dyadic (two people) setting or within a group can deliberately evoke recalling the past. It may be advisable to provide opportunities for both, as some residents may prefer one setting to the other. For reminiscence purposes, it can be more effective if the listener is female, and has had experience and training in active listening to encourage self-disclosure. Nonverbal research suggests that both females and males seem to prefer a female confidante. This is associated with the belief that women are more open and other-centered in their communication roles. Women are also viewed as being more reactive, supportive, and affiliative in their roles as speakers and listeners in conversation.

The value of reminiscence programming is immeasurable. Whenever possible, include a time for reminiscence with any other activities, even if it is a short discussion.

Chapter 11

INTERGENERATIONAL ACTIVITY

> The person who knows only her or his own
> generation remains forever a child.
> —Plato

A popular term that is related to activity programming for older citizens is "intergenerational." This includes bringing together individuals from different points on the life cycle to exchange views and learn to better understand each other. A successful project is described below:

REMEMBERING THE TEEN YEARS

If you want to know about the past, why not ask those who have directly participated in it? This was the premise of a team project that paired two high school students with a senior citizen in order to discover the similarities and differences about their teenage experiences.

"That's something I'll always have with me—my memories." A senior citizen is talking about his reaction to participation in an intergenerational project initiated by a local high school.

A series of three weekly interviews was scheduled with seniors living independently and those residing in a personal-care home. Students in the project were expected to hear responses from the seniors to a variety of prepared questions related to the older person's past. One of the project's goals was to result in an anecdotal but realistic record of the family life, social and work activities and school memories of the interviewees.

In order to accomplish this, a tape recorder was used for each session. As each interview was completed, students were expected to replay their tapes in order to index the content into major topic categories. Then the written index became a table of contents for future referral purposes when classroom assignments were associated with the interview material.

Since the high school class was English, students were to use the interviews as source material in order to create the following assignments:

- A character portrait of their senior citizen,
- A poem based on one of the experiences shared,
- A descriptive passage based on a discussion of the person's home place, and
- A short story which resulted from one of the many experiences the older person had shared with the students.

Each assignment was to be completed in consultation with the interviewee so that intergenerational team partnership could be strengthened.

The final segment of the project was the selection of the most effective pieces of writing. These were then edited and typed for publication as a source book, made available to all participants and any other interested community members. The book was placed in the school library and also presented to the local community library as an account of the teen experiences of the past.

The focus of the interviews was the teenage years of the senior citizens. Why was this specific topic chosen? It was considered to be a subject close to the immediate interests of the interviewers and one not so far from the interviewees' experience that they could view it with enthusiasm. Communication research suggests that self-disclosure elicits more self-disclosure. The interviews became a vehicle for enhancing communication opportunities between the two age groups.

Students were specifically asked to be the first to reveal personal information about their lifestyles as teenagers. In doing this, the older persons might hear something that would trigger earlier life memories of their own. For the most part, the communication technique was successful. Many seniors said how interesting it was to hear about the goings-on of the students. They served as reminders of their own years as teenagers, which they seemed very willing to share.

At first, most of the seniors were unfamiliar with their student interviewers and felt anxious about sharing personal information with strangers. To alleviate part of this discomfort, a group meeting was held just for the senior participants. At the meeting, a general outline of the project was presented and potential questions discussed. Approximately 30 seniors agreed to participate along with about 60 high school students. For the students, class lectures, written and oral interview guidelines and questions, and role-playing were presented to make them more competent oral interviewers.

A post evaluation of the project was given to both students and seniors. Twelve questions asked for responses to the structure and timing of the interviews, as well as the subject's satisfaction with the interview experience. In answer to the question, "What meant the most to you in this project?" some responses from the senior interviewees were:

- "It was so pleasant to remember and share."
- "I was glad to know that you are seeing the need for elder people's care and giving the young a chance to select us as their job, if they so wish."
- "Being able to let young persons know about the changes that have occurred and have an insight into people's lives before them."
- "Meeting interviewers and realizing that high school students of today aren't all bad."

In turn, selected student interviewer responses were as follows:
- "This helped me realize how important seniors felt during the talks and after them, and what experiences they were knowledgeable about."
- "Rather than trying to extract information from my person, I concentrated on making her feel appreciated."
- "I met an interesting man I learned a lot from."
- "I liked going through the years and struggles these people had to endure."
- "Having my senior say she loved us to death."

A young man wrote what meant the most to him during the interviews was "her smile. Kinda corny, huh?" Rather than corny, this project became one of the most meaningful the students had participated in all year.

Spending time with someone in our present day society is an indication of the interest you have in him or her. The more time you spend, the more interested you appear to be, and the reverse is equally revealing. Because a younger person seems to parcel out time more rigorously, the older person can appreciate the valuable time being given them by the young.

It is refreshing to observe the kind of project being described here, which highlights the advantages of pairing the adolescent with the senior citizen. Both have much to gain from each other. The younger person needs to have an image of what it feels like to be old, and the older person enjoys recapturing the exuberance of what it feels like to be young.

Rather than presenting one-time programs that provide momentary diversion for an older person's day, why not engage in the continuous sharing of memories which can provide ongoing lessons in understanding and learning from one another? So often we hear about generational conflict and misunderstanding between the young and old. What better way than reminiscing to find a common ground for sharing our most private possessions—our memories?

Bringing the generations together is a way to open up our lives to an awareness of other ages and experiences. If you have not tried intergenerational activities, here are some ideas to introduce the idea into your facility:

1. Find an intergenerational pen pal for residents and hold a monthly "pen pal day." You can also bring in letters from famous older people to read aloud and discuss, as a beginning.

2. Use a computer class to join older and young people—the young people can work to share their knowledge with the older people.

3. Watch a special television show or videotape with a younger person and have a discussion in a group.

4. Set up ongoing intergenerational projects and learning activities by matching different age groups together.

5. Create library days where elders are present in libraries to help young people find sources, discuss book problems, and enjoy literature.

6. School intergenerational day—Invite elders to take roles of "teachers-for-a-day" in classrooms, perhaps even on the University level.

7. College campuses - Schedule a nontraditional student day. Work with a university administrator or faculty as a liaison for setting it up. Have residents tour a campus or attend one or two classes for the day.

8. Organize an intergenerational Business Day in your community. Elders stay at a place of business for part of a day, either working or observing. At time's end, have them meet with employers, or complete an evaluation about their observations.

9. Family Days—Invite staff who have children, or residents' family members to share activities for the day.

10. Invite local schools to have a few residents as guest speakers on aging.

11. Invite civic clubs (Rotary, Kiwanis, etc.) to invite elders as guests, or as guest speakers on retirement, or on the value of intergenerational relationships.

12. Encourage international students or adults to share the way their culture regards aging and the elderly.

13. Make a quilt by requesting families, staff and residents to save large fabric pieces. Do this well in advance. Contact local quilters for assistance. Try having a quilter matched with each resident. Children might be invited to contribute squares of material and later in the project development, invite them as observers, or as helpers.

14. Invite storytellers as entertainment and have various ages in your audience.

15. Work up a talent show of residents, and invite children as the audience. First, have a resident explain to them how the show was created and have each "actor" introduced.

16. If a local drama person is available, a creative dramatization of an historical event of local or national interest might be rehearsed with an intergenerational cast of characters.

17. Plan an intergenerational panel discussion on a controversial national topic or a topic your residents' council suggests. Topics for consideration: community volunteerism, Saturday schooling, planning an intergenerational project/trip, having a fund raiser, importance of reading, evaluating television programs, how to choose gifts, etc.

18. Organize a People Scavenger Hunt by developing a list of traits and skills of people which participants have to discover in the other players. For example, list 10-20 items, depending on how many people participate. Consider different approaches: A team composed of an elder and a student, or individual players, or elders seeking younger people to identify and young people to find elders to identify. The winner matches the traits with people who have those traits. The objective is to encourage conversation between participants in order to find someone who has the trait or skill listed. All players should have their own list in bold-faced type with space to write-in the matching per-

son's first name, or initials. A prize can be given to the winning person or 2-person team working together.

Examples of Traits	Answers
1. Likes pizza	_____
2. July birthday	_____
3. Wears a hearing aid	_____
4. Favorite color - red	_____
5. Last name begins with "B"	_____
6. Speaks a foreign language	_____
7. Wears a birthstone	_____
8. Has four grandchildren	_____
9. Plays piano	_____
10. Went fishing	_____

Game: "What comes next?" Played with intergenerational groups. Index cards have lines of well-known slogans, quotes, songs, poems, or plots of familiar stories. One person draws a card and reads it aloud. Anyone in the group may fill in the next line. Examples can include:

"Tippecanoe and . . ."

"A penny saved . . ."

"It was many and many a year ago in a kingdom by the sea, lived a maiden there whom you may know by the name of . . ."

" . . .The young queen finally guessed the name of the dwarf as . . ."

Remember: Programs are limited only by your imagination! The best programs result from ideas expressed by getting diverse people together to "brainstorm." Ask, "If we want to get age groups together, what ideas do you have?"

or "What would residents enjoy working on with other age groups?"

Chapter 12

ART ACTIVITIES

The preacher visited the other day. He said I should be thinking of the here after. I told him, "Oh I do, all the time. No matter where I am I'm always asking myself: Now what am I here after?"
—Anonymous

Art is the creation of a person's vision. It is one of the oldest forms of human expression, which releases visual imagery formed in the mind of an individual. By varying materials and artistic tools, activities can stimulate and enrich the visual imagination. Adding music to art produces many favorable results. Consider the following ideas:

1. Residents can draw self-portraits with charcoal crayons, or pastels, or work with a partner they can sketch. Brown bags work well as materials or obtain large rolls of wrapping paper or white paper.

2. Trace the body silhouette of a partner lying on the floor, or trace the foot or hand of partner or self. Then color and cut out the silhouette. When finished, attach to wall with an adhesive double-sided tape, or put string through several cutouts, or affix with clothespins to a sturdy rope strung between two objects in a room. If both sides of cutouts are decorated, this makes an intriguing display. You can also cut out and decorate already drawn clothing items (shirts, coats, hats, aprons, etc.) and affix to body cutouts with tape or glue. If body silhouettes are too difficult, try sketching partner faces. Later, others can try to guess whose name goes with which face.

3. Using natural objects collected in association with the season (nuts, leaves, flower petals and stems, ferns, let-

tuce, beans, etc.) have residents arrange them in a tray, or on paper, with glue. Items can also be spray painted or decorated and colored with food coloring. Collages can also be made by cutting out magazine photos or greeting cards, or comic strip illustrations to create interesting "pictures," or original greeting or note cards.

4. Use textured rope or sponges dipped in dye or food coloring to create abstract designs when color—filled sponge rope is moved across paper.

5. With colored paper, already cut into shapes (abstract, geometrical, animal or birds) pair residents with partners who have chosen a like object shape. The shapes are then pasted/taped to paper and with drawing markers, residents add appropriate environments or objects on the page. Magazine illustrations of similar drawings could be made available to encourage ideas. (Example—bird in a nest, squirrel in a tree, ocean and a beach ball, etc.).

6. Invite local crafts or knitting instructors to provide a simple demonstration, to teach a new art skill to residents.

7. Using store-bought or hand-made flowers and small clay pots and ribbon, create artificial window pots for residents' rooms or public hallways.

8. Place three still-life objects on a table and invite residents to sketch them. When done, mount all attempts to encourage others to participate.

9. Using cloth napkins, demonstrate different ways to fold napkins and have residents replicate. You can place favors inside napkins or tie them with colored ribbons to use for actual mealtimes.

10. With tongue depressors (decorated or dipped in paint) attach ribbons, and paint or write names of residents. Use as bingo favors, or napkin accompaniment, or personal bookmarks.

11. Ask a local pizza place for boxes and cut out circles from each to fit different head sizes of residents. Next, staple fabric on circle "brim," or with crayons or brushes, paint

Art Activities

around brim to make decorative hats. Men can use wide brims with colored paper bag insets that fit into the middle of the brim. Finished hats can be displayed on a table or modeled by residents. Shirtfronts can also be made from pizza boxes, with string or ribbon holes attached on both sides to hold the shirt front in place around a male's chest.

12. Murals can help brighten drab rooms. Hospital patients and volunteers wielded their brushes at a "Paint-In" at Beth Israel Medical Center in Newark, New Jersey, in an effort to create cheerful murals. The event was part of a project by the Foundation for Hospital Art Inc., to encourage people to paint murals on hospital walls and ceilings. Can you think of a variation of this for your facility?

13. With colored nail polish or paint, decorate cutouts of silhouettes, of large-size fingernails or feet with toenails. They can then be mounted or mobiles made from them for room hanging decorations. For males, large cutouts of different fish, cars, sports objects or landscapes are interesting items to decorate.

14. Have residents create a sports wall mural. Supply appropriate cutout objects with double-sided tape which residents can add to a mural (baseball, bats, bags of peanuts, bases, and an uniformed team). Residents can decorate figures and sports area with color.

15. With sketches of sailboats already drawn or already cut out, decorate the sails and mount on a wall mural of brown paper. Make small boats out of paper and fill with candy or small items as table favors. You can use a nautical theme of "Row, Row, Row Your Boat" and other appropriate songs. Vote on the most attractive boat or other object created.

16. Ask local art teachers for a slide show of artists' works with accompanying commentary on each slide.

17. Contact a local art association to request several works to be exhibited and changed periodically in public areas of your facility.

18. Ask a local art association if members would come to demonstrate their art and involve residents in an art exercise or a project under their supervision.

19. Plan an intergenerational art project combining students, children, and your residents. Have a resident committee select a few ideas to consider.

20. With different dried beans and pebbles, fill empty food canisters. Make containers into rhythmic drums and create music by shaking or beating them. This is an easy way for arms and hands to be exercised and creates an energetic activity.

21. Ask local city council members to serve on an informal panel program to describe efforts to beautify the community and its landscaping, and solicit suggestions from residents. Take residents on a car or van tour to specific areas. The tour might elicit more suggestions.

22. Arrange a resident tour of a local museum, art gallery or special exhibit. Invite community persons as docents (knowledgeable tour guides).

23. With a collection of ribbons, bows, and package wrapping ornaments, have each resident attach their wrap ribbon to create a cardboard "bouquet," or make many bouquets to use as table centerpieces. Contact a department store to demonstrate effective gift box wrapping.

24. Create body chest banners out of wide ribbon or plastic strips. Decorate them with peoples' first names, initials, and decorated objects. These can be worn by residents or made for volunteers' identification for special occasions.

25. Invite Boy and Girl Scout troops to bring their models of hand-made cars or other craft items for display. Residents could vote on their favorites. Scouts can be asked to describe the task with questions encouraged from residents.

26. Through reminiscence activities, discuss interesting or significant events in residents' lives or in the facility. Then

select 5-6 items that can be drawn (either by staff, residents, or outside artists) on cardboard or as paper patterns. Have residents transfer the pattern, either with liquid crayons or other utensils to quilt or fabric pieces. The larger task is to sew quilt pieces together to create a wall hanging or individual quilted place mats. Family members can be encouraged to help.

27. Art Cutouts—You can create a colorful banner with felt cutouts of different animals, birds, or fish which can be attached to heavier fabric for wall banners or other decorative displays. Velcro is an easy attachment product for residents to work with, or try double-sided tape.

28. If a display board is available, draw shapes in large detail (triangles, circles, serpentine, etc.). A large piece of paper, adhesive-taped to the wall, will work well. The purpose of this activity is to encourage people to work together to think of many objects which have a particular shape. First, divide the group into pairs or small groups of three or four. (The larger the group, the easier it is to divide into small groups.) A director can begin by selecting and drawing the shapes, but as the activity progresses, encourage residents to take turns drawing a different shape each time. This helps stimulate visual memory. To make the game easier, specific categories could be suggested for each shape; i.e., "let's make these circles all edible" or "these should all be forms of transportation."

29. Card Talk—Just as some people enjoy saving attractive greeting cards, a collection of picture postcards from staff, families, and residents could be employed to introduce new scenic images to your residents. All cards are placed in a large box or basket and residents pick one. Each person's responsibility would be to describe the picture on the card to the rest of the group, and to connect the picture with a memory that the picture brings to mind. The card is then sent around the circle so that each person sees the picture.

30. Sand Art—Make simple trays filled with sand and place small items (knick-knacks, shells, twigs, buttons, or dolls) in trays. Each resident is invited to rearrange the items in a decorative manner. You can do the same with trays filled with yogurt, cool whip, sour cream, dough, etc., and practice making different designs with one utensil.

31. Tactile Objects—Collect old fabric samples from furniture, fabric or carpet stores. Blindfold residents and ask them to identify the "feel" of each, describing personal recollections from the different textures.

32. A Tactile Treasure Hunt—With wide-colored ribbon, string it either outside the facility or through several rooms, making the "scavenger" follow along the ribbon to touch hidden and/or numbered objects (fuzzy, smooth, prickly, felt, etc.) along the way. If done with a partner or in three's, one scavenger is blindfolded while the other two make sure their third person holds the ribbon to reach each hidden item.

33. Bag Masks—Create paper bag masks by working in pairs. Have already cut-out paper eyelash curls, string or ribbon hair decorations, and mustaches, paper eyes, nose, and lip cut-outs to be colored and attached to masks. Bag masks could be displayed on sticks or mounted on walls for public exhibit. Participants in drama activities (see next chapter) can also use these masks.

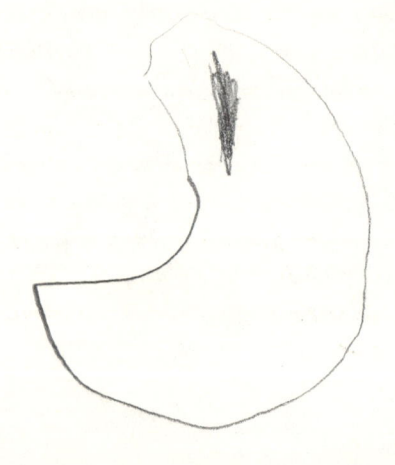

Chapter 13

DRAMA ACTIVITIES

God conceived the world, that was poetry;
He formed it, that was sculpture;
He colored it; that was painting;
He peopled it with living beings; that was the grand, divine, eternal drama."

—Charlotte Cushman

CREATIVE DRAMATICS AND PERFORMING

Creative dramatics is an improvisational strategy that frees the performer from memorizing the text, in order to focus on the individual's creative expression. Choose a single reminiscence, a published story, or familiar written text as an initial stimulus. The leader should make sure that everyone knows the story by first telling or reading it aloud to the group. Allow enough time for discussion and informal associations with the material. Each person is then asked her/his interpretation of the plot and what character they would like to portray. A major objective of creative dramatics is to permit a constant interchange of actors, so that everyone who desires to play a role is given the opportunity to do so. In this way, the dialogue remains fresh and varies with each new combination of actors. The leader's task is to divide the story into mini scenes; a new scene begins each time a character either enters or leaves the action.

Using creative dramatics techniques with elders is usually effective because there are no definite lines to remember. Spontaneous responses are often easier for many residents of long-term care settings who are troubled with memory deficits. Older performers are able to listen and respond spontaneously to other actors. There is no "right" way to act so every participant can put an individualized stamp on a scene. In many instances older people enjoy the rehearsal periods and the evaluations of presentations just as much as the actual performance itself. This is especially true when the material is drawn from their own personal narratives. For directors who prefer to use tailor-made scripts for older audiences, there are several sources available (e.g., *New Plays for Mature Actors*, 1989).

In England, several theatre groups combine their social service work for the elderly with performance interests. Transcripts of interviews conducted by "reminiscence workers" in the nursing homes are reworked into dramatic presentations. Scripts are based on specific time periods or influential events that are very familiar to elders of a specific geographic area. Examples of topics presented are seaside vacations, war memories and the London dock strike. Members of the cast are often elders themselves. Travelling reminiscence theatre groups travel the country, visiting areas noted for housing residential elder communities.

The highlight of a performance occurs before curtain time during the warm-up activity. Actors greet the audience informally and ask them to sing-along to music from the script's time period. Later, at the end of the play, a similar informal period is conducted, with all cast members seated in view of the audience. The cast invites the audience to comment on the ability of the script to capture memories from the audience's past. As Selzer (1986, p. 163) has written, "Memories float from us, like mists." Audience members may suggest additional reminiscences associated with the theme, which are then incorporated into subsequent performances. In this manner, the scripts are truly audience-created and audience-centered.

Program directors can use similar techniques to get residents thinking about the setting and evaluation of an activity before it actually begins. When people who participate in an activity are far fewer than the number who might appreciate being involved with it, a program director may have to spend additional time repeating it. It is suggested that those who initially took part will probably enjoy having another chance to present themselves before a larger group, to add to what was originally shared.

Although the greater proportion of older residents in long-term care is female, care should be taken to provide a balance of programs with appeal to both genders. There is a particular need to plan activities for which males play a prominent role. Besides asking residents for their suggestions, invite a male and a female to assume the positions of co-leaders of an activity program.

A Joke Contest works well. Have each participant rehearse at least one joke to share with a group. It is probably better to have no more than 4-5 jokesters at a time so that the judges' memories are not overloaded. In order to evaluate the audience's listening habits, ask a few people to try repeating a joke. If this proves difficult, allow the joker to serve as prompter, or have men and women work together as a team, practicing their oral presentation and dividing the presentation. Some jokes can be printed in a newsletter or shared orally during another occasion. A second time for presentation would give participants additional recognition and add much needed laughter into the environment. Laughter is healthy and needs to be encouraged in residential settings.

Masks—Providing unusual ways to express feelings can be achieved by working with residents to create or handle masks. Materials for masks can range from simple cardboard or fabric cutouts to elaborate paper maché creations. Masks allow people to take on a second identity. With the aid of masks, fables or familiar folk tales can be dramatized, along with personal narratives that residents wish to share. Residents can even be encouraged to use masks to represent various power figures in their lives (e.g., family members, residential staff, health professionals, and legal advisers). Listening to their improvised feeling-statements is both informative and therapeutic for all concerned.

An activity of this kind offers residents the opportunity to interpret themselves and their significant others. To facilitate handling, larger sized masks can be placed on a stand, or attached to a surface, so residents need only position themselves behind them. If masks are draped in black, actors wearing black clothing can sit directly behind the masks and appear to be giant puppet head figures. A narrator can also carry masks to the seated actors or even move among the audience to involve them more in the action. One caution: depending on the extent or intensity of the negative feelings—be prepared for emotional reactions from both performers, viewers, and listeners.

Words can be brought to life to heighten the dramatic imagination through pantomime, character portrayals, and role playing a situation or emotion and reading aloud. Drama techniques offer limitless opportunities for creative programming.

1. Situation Sources—Use everyday activities to discuss how residents view their life. Then role play one situation at a time. You may wish to be one of the leading characters, just to encourage the "actors." Role play the same situation several times with different people. Seek audience evaluation each time. (It is often easier to role play sources of daily conflicts that arise.)

2. Blindfold selected people, or have them use their hands up in front of their faces, and try to teach them a particular activity. This enhances their sensitivity to touch and commonplace situations.

3. You can experiment with voice communication (vocal loudness, softness, etc.) to simulate sensitivity to sounds.

Then conduct a discussion of people's comfort levels when voice changes occur.

4. Create a bingo-style pantomime game. If you land on certain squares, you must act out what it says. Examples: "I am grumpy," or "I can't find my key," "I am surprised!" etc.

5. Wishing—If you could become a well-known public figure, alive or dead, who would it be? Have residents make silent choices and then act out, or speak in the first person about their "wish person," suggesting clues so other residents can guess who it is. This can evoke other people's memories of the same well-known person.

6. Dramatize an emotion—Begin with a discussion of how moods and emotions affect us through the mind and the body. Follow this, by asking for suggestions of an emotion to dramatize. Choose one at a time and ask everyone to see how his or her body feels as you present a situation where that emotion is usually displayed. Talk about how positive emotions versus negative ones make us feel.

7. Hat Characters—Bring in a collection of hats. Have each resident choose one and talk about someone who might have worn it. Have them move, walk, or stand in a way the hat character might.

8. With a partner, mirror the emotions that a group leader orally calls out, to see how well you can match another person's facial expressions. Residents "become" each other's facial mirrors.

9. With a narrator reading a poem or singing lyrics, try to think of gestures that fit the words. Rehearse gestures several times for a voice or choral or movement activity.

10. Read aloud short scenes from plays. Enlarge the type and have enough copies for everyone. Exchange assigned parts often.

11. Using reminiscence stories from residents' past experiences, vote on one and then try dramatizing it.

12. Select a few situations (going on a picnic, plane travel, visiting a grandchild) and write a short radio play to dra-

matize. Tape record residents' reading the lines and exchange parts often. If individuals or the whole group wants to work on a script, take time to try out different lines. Eventually choose a few minutes to play the tape over the public address system. Residents may recall radio voices from the past like Fibber McGhee and Mollie, The Green Hornet, or Baby Snooks and use their character voices in common situations.

13. Poetry —Make copies of well-known poems or short rhymes or familiar song lyrics in LARGE PRINT. Practice reading aloud as a choral reading group, assigning specific lines to be spoken by individuals, or smaller groups of two and three. Keep going over and over the selections to polish the recitation. Add simple movements and group gestures and present as a program for others.

14. Plan a creative writing program: Bring in everyday objects as stimuli to write about. Talk about favorite poems and why you like them. Then, construct a *Group poem*:

(1) Use a blackboard or flipchart for group focus.

(2) Each person offers an image, word, phrase or line.

(3) A facilitator records them and reads them aloud.

(4) The leader keeps a meaningful message developing and as each idea is added the group puts a poem together.

15. Poetry— Read aloud famous poems or ask for recall of some. Ask each person to pick out favorite images or words. Discuss word associations and personal meanings associated with each. Collected poems of an author or anthologies are good sources.

16. Masking - Have residents sit and/or move about in a circle. One leader at a time calls out (or reads from a prepared slip of paper), "I am friendly . . .I am angry . . .I don't care . . .I am feeling badly," etc. The entire group must then convey the emotion announced. One person is chosen to decide on the next facial emotion until all emotions (on paper slips) are used.

17. Dress Up - Bring in hats, scarves (head and neck), hairpieces, and jewelry. With a Polaroid camera, take photos of dressed-up residents and post.

Chapter 14

MUSIC ACTIVITIES

What do you call music composed in bed? Sheet Music!!
—Anonymous

With either crayons or colored chalk, give each person a fairly large piece of blank paper. Use a tape recorder or a phonograph to play instrumental classical music that can evoke a strong mood. (If you need help with the selections, contact a local librarian.) These pieces can start you out: La Mer by Debussy, Gaite Parisienne by Offenbach, The Pines, or the Fountains of Rome by Resphiggi, The Swan from *Carnival of the Animals* by Saint Saens, The Triumphal March from Verdi's opera, *Aida*. Start off with a lively piece of music and then contrast it with a calmer, slower selection. For each selection, ask the participants to choose whatever color the music suggests to them. The more abstract the drawing the better.

The object of this exercise is to let the participants relax and be moved along by the sound and images the music creates. Each selection may be played twice, or as long as it takes for each person to finish a drawing. Sharing drawings with the group may take the form of silent recognition or verbal explanations of why people drew what they did. The director should ask how different pieces of music affect mood, and suggest different images that come to mind. It may be interesting to compare all the drawings created from one piece of music. This exercise can be varied by asking participants to use only certain kinds of strokes or certain colors for their drawing, or to use only certain areas of the paper.

The same music can become the stimulus for rhythmic movement exercises for certain body areas. This is especially important for patients in wheelchairs who do not have control of their total bodies. Talking about mental imagery that the music brings to mind can make it easier for a person to pretend that body parts can move like an object. "Your head is the strong wind, blowing the trees outside" or "Show me how your arms would move if they were the waves on a stormy day."

Music is therapeutic. By selecting music to change the mood, instrumental music can add to your residents' enjoyment. Try music at mealtimes. Be sure to ask for feedback from residents to determine whether or not this may be something you wish to continue.

Kitchen music—Borrow kitchen implements to distribute to residents for an activity. With an audiotape, a record, or instrument, select a piece with a strong rhythm and have residents accompany the song using the kitchen implements. At Christmas, buying different size bells for residents can be a fun way to "ring-along" with Christmas melodies. Some residents may find it easier to participate in this nonverbal way.

Music Memories—Secure and play recordings of old-time music. Have a reminiscence-guessing hour where residents must identify by name and/or sing along with the recorded music. Live music (piano, harmonica, etc.) is an even better substitute.

Add-a-Line—One person thinks of a line of a song. The final word of the line has to be picked up by someone who knows that word to be the first word of another line in a different song. For instance, "Let me call you sweetheart, I'm in love with *you*..." may lead to "*You* made me love you..." The exercise usually results in pleasant memories and group support.

Chapter 15

NATURE STIMULI ACTIVITIES

Most of us live ordinary lives and die ordinary deaths. But in the ordinary, there is a range of feelings and detail that is like the pattern in marble, only partly visible on the surface, but penetrating unseen into the body of the stone.
—Stephen Rosenfeld

Mother Nature may be the best teacher of all. Nature activities can include arranging direct experiences for residents with natural environments, handling objects, observations of nature's variations, and developing an awareness of selections and illustrations based on Nature's gifts. Bringing nature into your facility can be achieved with creative planning.

Nature and nature objects can be a source of interest and pleasure for older people. Bring nature's output into the facility to examine and discuss. Nature images can be compared with human behavior and life cycle stages. Here are some specific examples:

1. Collect leaves and place in groups in clear, plastic bags. Have residents trace around the boundaries with their fingers, comparing to the palms of their hands. Draw an outline of the leaf on paper.

2. Leaves can be pressed into clay or a like texture to examine leaf patterning.

3. Connect with stories of different uses for leaves, including using them as drinking cups when folded, leaves crushed or smoked for medicinal purposes, steamed or baked as part of a food source, used as transport or housing for imaginative "wee" characters in fantasy or children's literature.

4. Collect pussywillows and other dried flowers. Associate preserving pressed flowers and plants in books, with specific memories and potpourri uses.

5. Invite a florist, plant expert, or art teacher to demonstrate their methods. Have them bring along samples so residents can handle or create pressed flowers themselves.

6. With vegetable and flower seeds, show a stage-by-stage development and get seed pods for all residents to care for.

7. Using dried apples and other products, find a craftsperson who will demonstrate or teach "how to" use dried fruits as crafts.

8. Collect rocks from different areas and have a rock collector or geologist bring samples for everyone to handle. Add a quiz or contest to identify the rocks by type. Pair this activity with a guided tour of an area or a photo display of rocks.

9. Present a series of nature or outdoor slides and invite residents to offer their personal experiences and ideas about each one. Use as reminiscence "triggers" to elicit individual responses and recollections.

10. Distribute either the same fruit or flower or different fruits or flowers to everyone, have them draw the object from the outside, then from the inside (removing any outer covering or petals) examining the object in detail. Discuss the final evolution of the object as it begins from a seed.

11. Check video stores for travel films and any documentaries about natural earth movements.

12. Schedule a group television viewing of a nature program, and have a discussion of the program topic.

AFTER WORDS

This book is intended to provide fresh thoughts and new insights to apply to long-term care. The greatest contribution you can make to the lives of older people is to give of yourself, in the form of a sincere interest and responsiveness toward them and through the creative enthusiasm and involvement brought to activity programming.

Treat each day as an opportunity to try a different approach to your facility's communication activities. Keep this book within easy reach to remind you of the multiple choices available in activity programming. Though the work you do is need-driven, it also contributes significantly to the well being of older residents under your care.